THE DIABETES HANDBOOK

Non-insulin Dependent
Diabetes

THE DIABETES HANDBOOK
Non-insulin Dependent Diabetes

Dr. John L. Day M.D.,F.R.C.P.

THORSONS PUBLISHING GROUP
Wellingborough · New York

Published in collaboration with
The British Diabetic Association
10 Queen Anne Street, London W1M 0BD

British Library Cataloguing in Publication Data

Day, John L.
    The diabetes handbook.
    Non-insulin dependent diabetes
    1. Diabetes — Treatment   2. Self-care,
    Health
    I. Title   II. British Diabetic Association
    616.4'6206   RC660

    ISBN 0-7225-1369-0

Printed and bound in Singapore

Contents

Foreword

Today people with diabetes can lead full and active lives and expect to be as healthy as people without diabetes. However, to enjoy good health with diabetes demands self-discipline, understanding and knowledge. Nobody can be expected to follow rules and recommendations without a clear explanation of the reasons for doing so.

So it is a pleasure to welcome this new British Diabetic Association Handbook. It is comprehensive and thoroughly up-to-date. It contains all the essential information.

The Handbook has been prepared by experts in the field. It is clearly and sympathetically written, copiously illustrated and well designed, so that even the most complex aspects of diabetes and its control are easy to understand. It is invaluable as a reference book and as an easy to follow practical guide to good diabetic control. Nobody with diabetes should be without it.

Sir Harry Secombe CBE

Introduction

History

The correct name for diabetes is diabetes mellitus. 'Diabetes' is derived from a Greek word meaning syphon, and 'mellitus' refers to the characteristic sweetness of the urine of people with diabetes. This title describes one of the most important features of the disease — the passage of very large amounts of sweet urine.

Diabetes is very common. In the UK there are more than 600,000 people with diabetes, of whom over 30,000 are children; worldwide there are over 30 million.

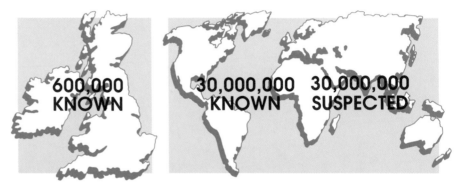

Fig. 1.1
The estimated numbers of people with diabetes.

Diabetes has been known to physicians for thousands of years, one of the first references to it being in the Ebers Papyrus (Fig. 1.2) written in Egypt in 1500 BC. It is also referred to in ancient Indian, Roman, Japanese and Chinese writings. However, it was not until the last century that any significant advance was made in understanding the nature of diabetes, or in developing an effective form of treatment. The first major breakthrough came in 1889, when two German scientists discovered that the removal of the pancreas, a large gland in the abdomen, gave rise to diabetes. About this time, it was also discovered that damage to specific cells in the

Fig. 1.2
The Ebers Papyrus.

Written about 1500 BC, this is one of the earliest documents describing the treatment of diabetes. The treatment is called "A medicine to drive away the passing of too much urine . . ." and included a mixture of bones, wheat grains, fresh grits, green lead, earth and water. These ingredients the user should "let stand moist, strain it, take it for four days."

The Payprus, measuring over 20 metres long and 30 centimetres wide, was found in a grave in Thebes in Egypt, in 1862.

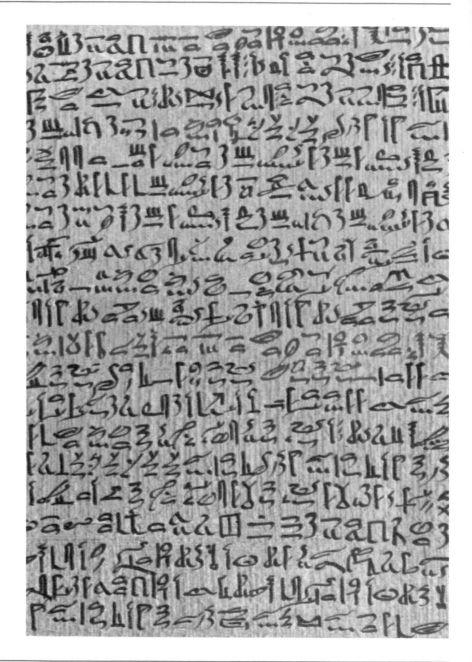

pancreas, called islets of Langerhans, produced certain forms of diabetes. But it was not until 1921 that two Canadians, Frederick Banting and Charles Best (Fig. 1.3) made their famous discovery of insulin.

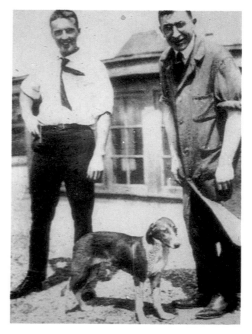

Fig. 1.3
Banting and Best.
Frederick Banting and Charles Best, whose research led to the isolation of insulin. The photograph shows them with their famous dog, Marjorie, which was kept alive by insulin after her pancreas had been removed.

Modern treatment enables many thousands of people with diabetes to achieve complete, fruitful, healthy lives and to fulfil their ambitions in all walks of life. Treatment is a bar to very few jobs. People with diabetes are found amongst our most successful actors, actresses, entertainers, politicians, first-class footballers, sportsmen and sportswomen competing at the highest level, and in all the professions; all of these bear witness to the fact that effective treatment can be combined with the highest achievements.

What is diabetes?

In simple terms, diabetes is a disorder in which the body is unable to control the amount of sugar in the blood, because the mechanism which converts sugar to energy is no longer functioning properly. This leads to an abnormally high level of sugar in the blood, which gives rise to a variety of symptoms initially and, if uncontrolled over several years, may damage various tissues of the body. Therefore,

How does diabetes develop?

the treatment of diabetes is designed not only to reverse any symptoms you might have at the beginning, but also to prevent any serious problems developing later.

Normally, the amount of sugar (glucose) in the body is very carefully controlled. We obtain sugar from the food we eat, either from sweet things, or after the digestion of starch foods (carbohydrates), such as bread and potatoes. Under certain circumstances, however, sugar can be made in the body by breaking down body stores. This will occur when the food supply is reduced, or when more sugar is needed, such as following an injury or during an illness.

The conversion of sugar to energy requires the presence of the hormone insulin, which is produced by the pancreas. Insulin is released when the blood sugar rises after a meal, and its level falls when the blood sugar decreases (Fig. 1.4), for example during exercise. Therefore, it can be seen that insulin plays a vital role in maintaining the correct level of blood sugar, particularly by preventing the blood sugar from rising too high. When there is a shortage of insulin, or if the available insulin does not function correctly, then diabetes will result.

Fig. 1.4
Blood sugar and insulin levels rise and fall after each meal or snack.

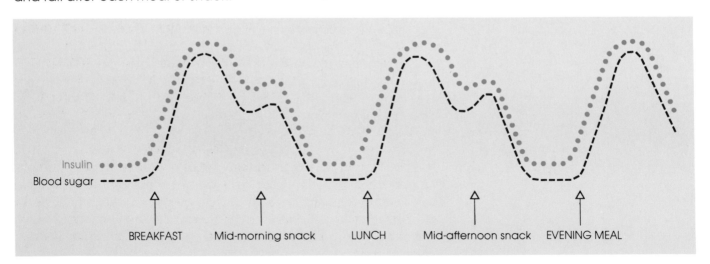

Insulin ● ● ● ●
Blood sugar ‑ ‑ ‑ ‑

BREAKFAST · Mid-morning snack · LUNCH · Mid-afternoon snack · EVENING MEAL

The consequences of diabetes are summarized below:

1. Because the blood sugar is not converted to energy, the amount of sugar in the blood builds up and spills into the urine.
2. In an attempt to compensate for the lack of energy, the liver makes much more sugar than normal.
3. Since there is an inadequate amount of insulin to convert the sugar to energy, another energy source has to be found. The body's stores of fat and protein are therefore broken down to release more sugar into the bloodstream, and there is a consequent loss of weight.
4. In the complete absence of insulin, the breakdown of fats may be excessive and substances called ketones — the breakdown products of fatty acids — will be found in the blood and will spill into the urine.

Somes ketones are acids, and if very large amounts are present, as for example in severe insulin deficiency, they cause the very serious condition of diabetic keto-acidosis or diabetic pre-coma.

Type of diabetes

There are two main types of diabetes:

1. Non-insulin dependent diabetes — also known as Type II diabetes or maturity onset diabetes.
2. Insulin dependent diabetes — also known as Type I diabetes or juvenile diabetes.

The essential difference between these two types is that people with insulin dependent diabetes, because they produce little or no insulin, will not survive unless they are treated with insulin. This is exactly what happened to people with diabetes before insulin treatment started in 1922.

In non-insulin dependent diabetes insulin is still produced, although it may be in inadequate amounts, or it may not be working properly. These people do not need insulin in order to survive and, in most cases, can be effectively treated by diet, or by a combination of diet and tablets. Only rarely do people with non-insulin dependent diabetes require insulin in order to establish perfect control.

The causes of diabetes and who gets it

In the United Kingdom, as many as 1 to 2 per cent of the population, and perhaps one in every 500 schoolchildren, have diabetes. It can occur at any age, but it is very rare in infants and becomes much commoner in the middle and older age groups. Amongst younger people, the sexes are almost equally affected by diabetes, whereas in older age groups, diabetes is commoner in women.

Non-insulin dependent diabetes

Cause

In this type of diabetes there is some insulin in the body, but not enough to maintain good health. The cause is not known.

Who gets it?

Non-insulin dependent diabetes used to be called 'maturity onset diabetes', indicating that it occurs in the middle and older age groups, although it occasionally occurs in young people. Overweight people are particularly likely to develop this type of diabetes, as are members of certain families in whom the condition is passed from one generation to the next.

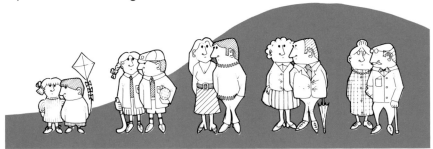

Insulin dependent diabetes

Cause

In this type of diabetes there is a complete or near complete absence of insulin, due to destruction of the insulin-producing cells of the pancreas. There is some tendency for insulin dependent diabetes to run in families, but the condition is far from being entirely inherited. The exact cause of the damage to the insulin-producing cells is not known for certain, but a combination of factors may be involved including:

- Damage to the insulin-producing cells, as a result of viral and other infections
- An abnormal reaction of the body against the insulin-producing cells.

Who gets it?

In general, younger people with diabetes (less than 40 years of age) are usually insulin dependent, but all age groups, even the very old, may be affected.

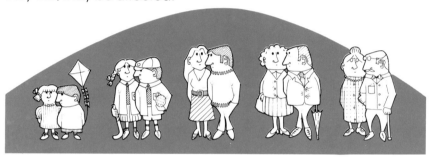

Other causes of diabetes

Diseases of the pancreas

A very few cases of diabetes are due to various diseases of the pancreas, such as inflammation of the pancreas (pancreatitis), or unusual deposits of iron. Occasionally, it occurs in rare forms of hormone imbalance.

Accidents or illnesses

Major accidents or illnesses are not thought to cause diabetes but, by causing a temporary increase in blood sugar, they may reveal pre-existing clinical diabetes, or make worse established diabetes. If your diabetes was discovered during the course of an illness, it is highly likely that you had diabetes before the illness, even though you did not show any symptoms.

Occasionally, during very severe illnesses such as a coronary, serious injury, or after a major operation, the blood sugar may rise, producing a state of temporary diabetes.

Psychological stress is not believed to cause diabetes, but may certainly exacerbate it.

Drugs

Some drugs can increase the blood sugar and may reveal pre-existing diabetes. Cortisone-like (steroid) drugs commonly do this, while water tablets (diuretics), which eliminate fluid from the body, do so less commonly. There are no other commonly used drugs which have this effect.

The contraceptive pill

The oral contraceptive pill does not cause diabetes, but it may raise the blood sugar slightly in those who already have the condition.

Heredity

Hereditary factors have already been briefly mentioned. The risk that the child of a father or mother who takes insulin may develop some type of diabetes before 20 years of age is higher than normal, but is still very small, probably about 1 per cent. In the rare situation where both parents have this type of diabetes the risk is further increased, but by an uncertain amount, and in such cases professional genetic counselling may be sought.

In the more common, non-insulin dependent diabetes, the situation is somewhat different, in that the condition is predominantly inherited. Because this type of diabetes usually occurs in people who are middle-aged or older, there are relatively few women of child-bearing age with non-insulin dependent diabetes.

So, to summarize, it is possible for someone to inherit a proneness to diabetes, but not the condition itself, which will only develop as a result of the influence of some other factor. Thus, there are a large number of people who never develop diabetes, even though they have an inherited tendency to do so.

Onset of symptoms and their severity

The main symptoms of diabetes are:

- Thirst and a dry mouth
- Passing large amounts of urine
- Weight loss
- Tiredness
- Itching of the genital organs
- Blurring of vision.

Symptoms vary considerably in their severity and rate of onset.

Non-insulin dependent diabetes

The symptoms develop more gradually and are usually less severe than in insulin dependent diabetes. Diabetic coma does not occur in this type of diabetes.

Some people fail to notice any symptoms, but after being treated they usually have more energy and feel considerably better. Unfortunately, the presence of symptoms is no guide to the level of sugar in the blood, and it is essential that diabetes is treated, even when there are no symptoms.

During an illness, usually an infection such as a chest or urinary infection, the symptoms of non-insulin dependent diabetes may worsen. In such instances, routine treatment by diet alone may prove inadequate, and tablets or insulin may prove necessary temporarily.

Insulin dependent diabetes

The condition develops fairly quickly, usually over a few weeks, but it may take as little as a few days, or as long as several months. Without insulin treatment the condition progressively worsens, resulting in a significant weight loss, dehydration, vomiting, the onset of drowsiness, and diabetic coma.

Treatment

Diabetes is a very common disorder. **Although no 'cure' is possible, all types of diabetes can be treated and normal health restored.**

Treatment is with:

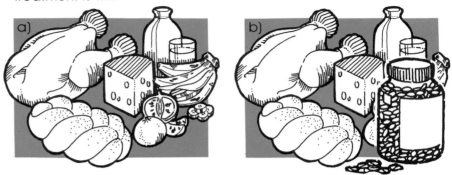

● Diet or diet and tablets — for non-insulin dependent diabetes

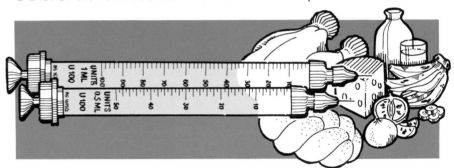

● Insulin and diet — for insulin dependent diabetes.

Treatment must be maintained throughout life. This is necessary not only to avoid symptoms and the risk of coma, but also to minimize the risks of any later complications.

Both forms of treatment require some modification to daily routines, and the performance of checks to ensure that treatment is effective. However, you should be able to achieve these with only minimal disturbance to your daily life.

From Chapter 2 onwards, this Handbook explains in detail what has gone wrong in your type of diabetes and describes how, with correct treatment, you should be able to maintain effective control.

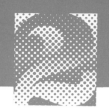

Non-insulin dependent diabetes

To understand the causes of non-insulin dependent diabetes, and to appreciate how you can manage your treatment, it is necessary to know some basic facts about the food you eat, how it is broken down in the body, how it is used and what may have gone wrong to cause your diabetes.

Some basic facts about nutrition

Our food is made up of three basic types — carbohydrates, fats and proteins, all of which are essential for a balanced diet (Fig. 2.1). As Fig. 2.2 shows, these three types of food are broken down by digestive processes in the intestinal tract and absorbed into the blood stream. For example, carbohydrates — the starchy foods, such as bread and potatoes — are broken down and converted to simple sugars, such as glucose, by the digestive juices of the mouth, stomach and intestines. The breakdown products of digestion are then absorbed into the blood stream and carried to the individual body cells. Fig. 2.2 shows that sugars and fatty acids provide energy, while amino acids, often referred to as the body's 'building blocks', are used to build cells and tissues and in excess are converted to glucose.

Fig. 2.1
Carbohydrates, fats and proteins are essential for a balanced diet.

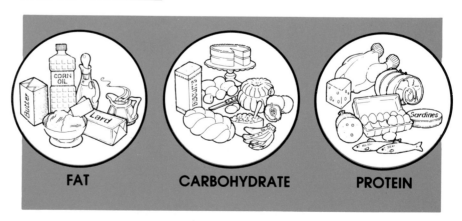

FAT   CARBOHYDRATE   PROTEIN

The whole process of food breakdown and usage, and the excretion of waste products, is termed metabolism. Metabolism is extremely complex, and in the healthy individual is very finely balanced, so that the body functions smoothly. Any imbalance in the metabolism of one type of food produces an effect on the metabolism of other types of food. For example, if the body is unable to convert sugar to energy, then the metabolism of fat and protein will be affected. In fact, this is exactly what happens in diabetes.

What has gone wrong?

In Chapter 1 the role of sugar control in the development of diabetes was briefly considered, and it is now appropriate to examine the significance of sugar metabolism in more detail. A basic knowledge of sugar metabolism is the key to understanding diabetes, so it is worthwhile carefully reading and re-reading the next few pages until the process is clear in your mind.

Where does blood sugar come from?

In the healthy individual, the level of blood sugar is kept within close limits, but will obviously be at its lowest several hours after a meal, and at its highest just after a meal. Under normal circumstances, the main source of blood sugar is the food we eat:

- **Sweet things** e.g. sugar added to cereals, drinks, sweets, jams, etc.
- **Starch foods** e.g. bread, potatoes, cereals, flour, etc.
- **Other foods** e.g. protein, may be converted to glucose.

Fig. 2.2 shows that sugar is absorbed into the blood supply and is transported to the individual body cells, where it is used for the production of energy. Excess sugar is converted to fat (triglyceride) and stored in the fat stores of the body, or it is converted to starch (glycogen), which is stored in the liver, for use as an energy supply in time of need. Eating too much overall increases the blood sugar and the weight.

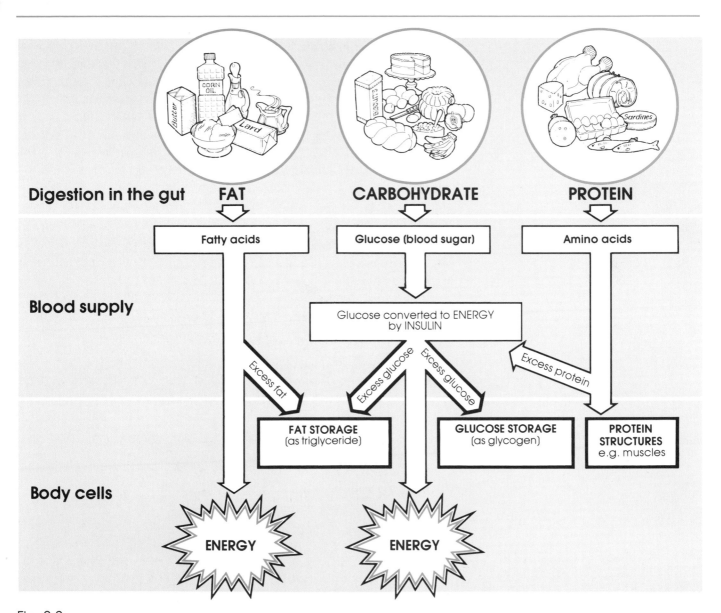

Fig. 2.2
Normal metabolism.
In the presence of insulin, glucose can be converted to energy.

The role of insulin

The key to the conversion of sugar to energy, or its storage as starch and fat, is insulin. Insulin, however, not only enables sugar to be converted to energy but also helps to increase the amount of stored energy, by preventing excessive breakdown of fat.

Insulin is produced by the pancreas, a gland situated at the back of the abdomen, and having the structure shown in Fig. 2.3. The pancreas is able to sense the level of blood sugar, and when this rises it will push more insulin into the circulation. Thus, the level of insulin is highest just after a meal and lowest when fasting or during exercise (Fig. 2.4). In your type of diabetes, although you are producing insulin, the supply is insufficient to cope with demand

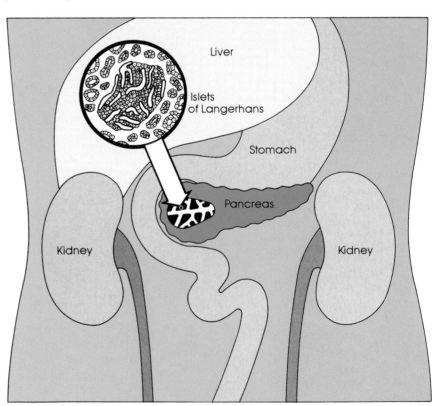

Fig. 2.3
The pancreas.
The pancreas is a large gland positioned behind the stomach. The inset shows the detailed structure of the insulin-producing cells, the islets of Langerhans.

Fig. 2.4
Insulin released from the pancreas makes the blood sugar level fall.

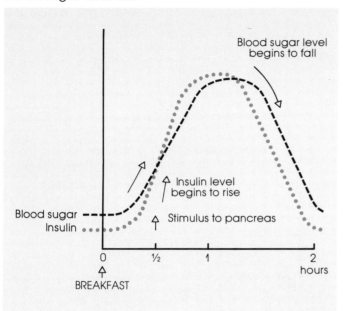

Fig. 2.5
In diabetes, insufficient insulin results in an excessively high blood sugar.

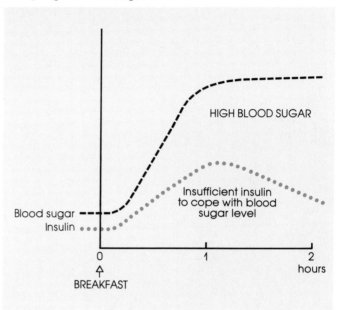

and this leads to a partial failure in the conversion of blood sugar to energy (Fig. 2.5). As you eat, therefore, the sugar level in the blood increases to a higher than normal level (hyperglycaemia). This is the hallmark of diabetes — an excessively high blood sugar.

Who gets diabetes and why?

There may be two contributory factors to the development of your diabetes:

1. The pancreas may produce enough insulin, but it does not work effectively.

2. The pancreas may be unable to produce enough insulin to maintain the blood sugar within the normal range.

Non-insulin dependent diabetes occurs in various groups of individuals:

- It occurs most commonly in people who are overweight. The reason for this is that fat tissue interferes with the action of insulin, so that overweight people need considerably more insulin than normal individuals. If, in addition, an overweight person has a less than normal production of insulin, because of a defect in the pancreas, then clearly the supply of insulin will be insufficient to prevent the development of diabetes. Also, because some overweight people tend to over-eat, the supply of sugar may be too high to be processed by the available insulin. In most cases, this type of diabetes can be readily controlled by simply eating less and losing weight, thereby allowing the insulin to work more effectively.

- This type of diabetes also occurs in people who are not overweight but who produce inadequate amounts of insulin.

- Some people are predisposed to diabetes by a tendency to be unable to produce enough insulin. This tendency may only become obvious at times when more sugar than normal is required, such as during an illness or after injury. It is important to stress that injury or illness are not believed to cause the diabetes, but rather they make it more obvious.

- In a few families, there is a strong hereditary element, and diabetes may be passed from generation to generation.

- It appears to be more common in some parts of the world, such as South America or Malta, than others, for example, Alaska.

Symptoms of high blood sugar

Sugar in the urine

As the blood sugar rises above normal, there comes a point when it begins to spill over into the urine (glycosuria).

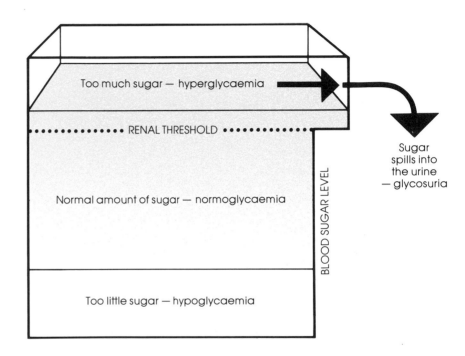

Too much sugar — hyperglycaemia

RENAL THRESHOLD

Normal amount of sugar — normoglycaemia

BLOOD SUGAR LEVEL

Too little sugar — hypoglycaemia

Sugar spills into the urine — glycosuria

Fig. 2.6
Blood sugar levels.
When the blood sugar reaches a certain level it spills over into the urine.
This level is called the renal threshold.

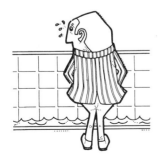

Usually, no sugar appears in the urine, unless the kidneys are malfunctioning. In a person with diabetes, however, the excess sugar is allowed to pass into the urine (Fig. 2.6), and this gives rise to three of the commonest symptoms of diabetes:

● **Passing large quantities of urine**
In order to get rid of the excess sugar, more water is excreted by the kidneys, and this results in the frequent passing of large volumes of urine. It may cause bed-wetting in some children, and incontinence in the elderly.

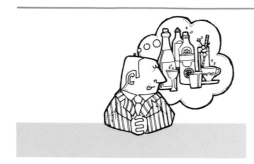

● Thirst

Because more water is leaving the body, the mouth becomes dry and thirst develops. The sensation may be so intense and disagreeable that sometimes even talking and swallowing become difficult. Soft drinks which contain a lot of sugar should be avoided, because they actually increase the blood sugar, resulting in an even greater thirst.

● Genital soreness

When a large quantity of sugar is passed in the urine, it tends to cause irritation around the genital area, and thrush may develop. It frequently causes itching of the vulva in women and, less frequently, itching of the penis in men. However, once diabetes is controlled and sugar disappears from the urine, these problems usually disappear.

Breakdown of body energy stores

Because a shortage of insulin means that the blood sugar cannot be converted into energy, energy must be provided from elsewhere. Consequently, there is a breakdown of fat and protein which results in:

● Weight loss

Diabetes is one of the commonest causes of weight loss. This occurs in most people with diabetes at the onset of the disorder. It ranges from a few pounds to 2 or 3 stone. Appetite is commonly unaffected and may even be increased, but not everyone loses weight, so do not ignore other symptoms.

● Tiredness and weakness

Tiredness, often accompanied by a sensation of weakness, is very common in uncontrolled diabetes. Some people are more than usually prone to fall asleep at odd times, while others just feel they are growing old before their time. This symptom can be readily reversed by treatment. Many feel 'rejuvenated' after treatment, even when they had previously been unaware of any abnormalities.

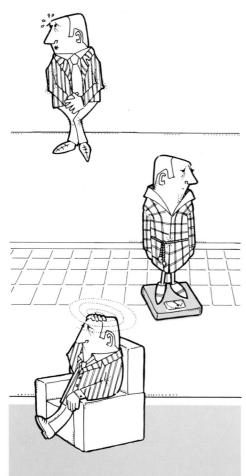

Other effects of high blood sugar

These include:

● **Blurring of vision**
The high level of sugar in the body causes the lens of the eye to change slightly in shape. Some people with diabetes become short-sighted when they first develop the disorder, but the reverse sometimes occurs, making reading difficult. These changes may only be noticed in the early stages of the treatment, and normally the ability to focus is completely restored in two or three weeks. It is wise, however, not to have your eyes tested for at least two months after proper stabilization of the diabetes.

● **Excessive loss of fluid/diabetic coma**
It is important to stress that in your type of diabetes, the so-called 'diabetic coma', which results from an extremely high blood sugar level, does not occur. Very rarely, if a vomiting illness, such as gastroenteritis, coincides with the development of your diabetes, then the blood sugar level may become unusually high. This can cause a significant increase in fluid loss, which may require hospital treatment. If you are eating normally, however, excessive fluid loss should not occur.

Symptomless diabetes

Most people with diabetes are aware of symptoms when the blood sugar is very high, but others may be quite unaware of their condition. For instance, diabetes is often detected at a routine medical examination for insurance employment purposes, or during an investigation of some quite unrelated illness.

Long-term effects of high blood sugar

If the blood sugar remains high for a period of years — even if it is not causing symptoms — it may cause damage. Particularly common are: damage to the small blood vessels in the feet; damage to the small nerves, creating a tingling sensation in the feet; or the development of a cataract. Early, effective treatment of diabetes should prevent these from developing. Where they have already developed, the sooner they are detected, the more effective will be their treatment.

Complications of diabetes are considered in more detail in Chapter 5, page 63.

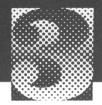

Treatment

Aims of treatment

There are two main aims of treatment:

1. Eliminate symptoms

The high blood sugar level is largely responsible for the symptoms of diabetes. Therefore, the first aim of treatment is to reverse any symptoms you might have, by returning the blood sugar level to normal. Once treatment has started, your feeling of well-being will be restored, any tendency to develop infections will be minimized, and, as long as treatment is continued, there should be no recurrence of symptoms.

2. Prevent late complications

If a high blood sugar is maintained over many years, then the eyes, kidneys and small nerves to the feet may be damaged. Clearly, there is every reason for returning your blood sugar level to normal and, by keeping to your treatment, reducing the risk of these complications.

IT IS IMPORTANT THAT YOU CONTINUE WITH YOUR TREATMENT, EVEN WHEN THE SYMPTOMS HAVE GONE, AND THAT YOU UNDERGO REGULAR CHECKS TO ENSURE THAT YOUR CONTROL IS BEING MAINTAINED.

The steps you need to take

Diet

● **Reduce your weight**

Most people with non-insulin dependent diabetes are overweight, and therefore the most important measure needed to control blood sugar levels is to reduce weight by dieting, and then to maintain it at the desired level. Your aim should be to reach a point where the insulin you produce is able to maintain your blood sugar at a normal level.

- **Control your sugar intake**

  This means avoiding or reducing the amount of those foods in the diet which lead to a rise in blood sugar, particularly sweets and refined sugars.

- **Reduce your fat intake**

  Cut back on fats and fatty foods if you are overweight.

- **Balance your diet**

  It is important that you ensure that the food you eat provides the right balance, so that you not only avoid those items which increase the blood sugar, but also an excess of other foodstuffs which might cause damage in other ways.

All of these essential adjustments to your diet can be achieved fairly easily, and you can continue to eat interesting and pleasant food.

Exercise

If you are able, it is important that you should take regular exercise. This will not only help to keep your blood sugar low but, if you are overweight, will also help you reduce your weight.

Other treatment measures

- **Tablets**

  If the above measures prove inadequate, you may be advised to take some special tablets to increase the efficiency of your diet.

- **Insulin injections**

  Insulin injections are not required, except occasionally when all the above measures have proved unsuccessful.

DIET

Let us now consider the importance of diet in more detail. To help you find a balanced diet which will enable you to control your diabetes, it is necessary to understand the basic facts about food and how it is broken down and used by the body.

The basic components of food

As outlined in Chapter 2, page 11, our food is made up of three basic types, namely carbohydrates, proteins and fats, all of which are essential for a balanced diet. Many foods contain mixtures of one or more types. For example, milk is made up of carbohydrate, protein and fat, eggs contain fat and protein, and pastry is mainly fat and carbohydrate. In general, vegetables and fruit contain little or no fat, while cheese, margarine and meat contain no carbohydrate.

Carbohydrate

Carbohydrate is found in:

● Sweet foods, such as sugar, jams and sweetened manufactured foods (Fig. 3.1)
● Starch foods, such as potatoes, cereal and pastry (Fig. 3.2)
● Some fruit and vegetables (Fig. 3.2).

Fig. 3.1
Carbohydrates: some typical foods containing large amounts of sugar.

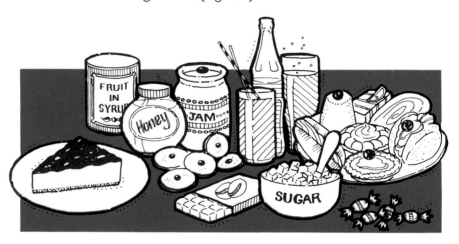

23

Fig. 3.2
Carbohydrates: some typical
starch-containing foods.

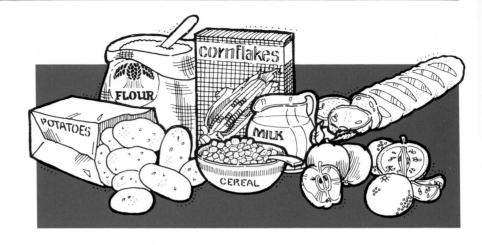

Protein

Protein is provided in such foods as meat, eggs, fish (Fig. 3.3), dairy products and some vegetables. Some protein in the diet is essential, because it provides the building materials for the cells and tissues of the body.

Fig. 3.3
Common foods containing mainly protein.

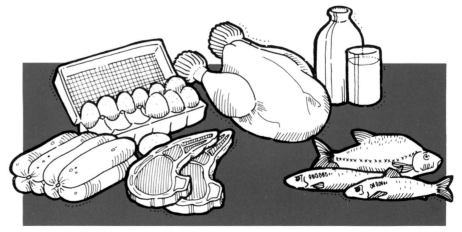

Fat

As well as obvious sources of fat (Fig. 3.4), such as butter, margarine, oil, lard and dripping, most meats, dairy products and eggs contain fat. Because even small amounts of fat contain a large number of calories, only small quantities are absolutely necessary for the maintenance of good health.

Fig. 3.4
Common foods containing a lot of fat.

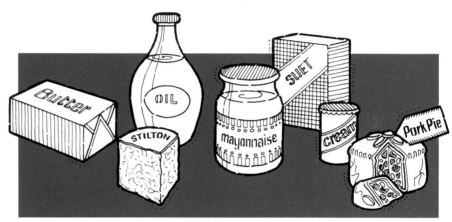

Other important components of the diet

These include:

Minerals and vitamins

With the right balance of carbohydrate, protein and fat, minerals and vitamins will be automatically included and supplements will not be necessary.

Fibre

This provides much of the bulk in most vegetables and some fruit, and is present in large quantities in unrefined cereal. Unfortunately, much of the fibre may be removed during modern food processing, a good example being the making of white flour and the milling of rice. Fibre is particularly valuable in diabetes, as it moderates the absorption of food.

Which foods should you eat?

The foods you eat should be determined by your weight. The diet for people with diabetes who are overweight is somewhat different from that for those with diabetes who are of normal weight. But, whatever your weight, you should avoid all very sweet foods and drinks, which cause a rapid rise in blood sugar.

If you are overweight, you should read the next section (light blue pages); if, however, your weight is normal, you should turn to the section beginning on page 35.

DIET IF YOU ARE OVERWEIGHT

Principles

The adjustments to your diet are based on the following two principles:

1. Avoid very sweet foods and drinks (Table 1), thereby minimizing the amount of sugar which has to be disposed of by your reduced insulin supply.

TABLE 1 Foods to be avoided

The foods listed below are high in sugar and have virtually no nutritional value:

Marmalade*/jam*/honey*/mincemeat/lemon curd
Golden syrup/black treacle
Sugar/glucose/glucose tablets
Fizzy and mixer drinks*, cordials* and squashes*, unless marked 'no sugar'/'low calorie'.
Bottled sauces and chutneys (in large amounts)
Buns/pastries/sweet biscuits
Sweets and chocolates
Fruit tinned in syrup*
*Low-sugar alternatives are available.

2. <u>Lose weight by reducing your intake of all those foods which provide energy in excess of your requirements</u>, so that your body will be forced to burn off its own fat. In other words, you will have to eat less food — particularly fats and sugary carbohydrate. Your dietitian or doctor will calculate how much food you will require to provide a balanced diet, supply sufficient energy, and allow you to lose weight. Very often a calorie allowance will be suggested.

Once you have reached your desired weight, your diet will be altered to that suitable for a person of normal weight. <u>However, it is important that your weight remains constant</u>, so make regular checks and if your weight increases, cut back as previously advised.

Some basic facts

Losing weight is never easy, particularly at first, but the more you know about foods and diet, the better you will be able to cope.

- Different people need different amounts of food. It may seem unfair that, even though you are already eating less than a slim person, you are still overweight. However, the fact remains that, in order to lose weight, you will need to eat less food than your body needs, thereby causing you to burn up your own excess fat.

  A good guide to start with is to avoid fatty and sugary foods as much as possible, and to have smaller quantities of food at each meal.

- It takes time to become overweight, so you should not expect to lose weight very quickly. A loss of one or two pounds (one kilogram) a week is perfectly adequate. At first, you may lose weight faster, perhaps as much as three quarters of a stone (5-6 kilograms) in the first month, but subsequently your weight loss will probably slow down. Do not become discouraged — continue with the diet until it shows the final results that you are aiming for.

- Many people believe that some foods are slimming and others fattening. This is not strictly true, since all foods, if taken in the wrong amounts, can cause problems. Therefore, it is important to learn which foods will help you to lose weight, how much of each you can eat at any one time, and also the best way of cooking each type of food.

● A restriction of fluid intake is sometimes advised, because excess fluid is often blamed for weight gain. This is quite unnecessary, however, and a normal intake of fluid is recommended, taking care to avoid sweetened or malted drinks.

Some dietary guidelines

To help you decide what to eat in order to ensure balanced, nutritious meals, but at the same time control your calorie intake, we have divided the various foods into four main groups:

1. Carbohydrate starch foods

2. Dairy products

3. Protein and fat foods

4. Fruit and vegetables.

Carbohydrates

● This groups includes flour, bread, pasta, rice, potatoes and breakfast cereals, as well as sweet foods which should, of course, be avoided (Fig. 3.5).

● This is one of the most important groups in your weight-reducing diet, and at least three small helpings from this group should be taken every day. A complete list is given in Appendix 2, page 99.

● You cannot and must not try to control your diabetes by avoiding starch foods altogether, but some limitation will be necessary.

● Recent evidence has indicated that the best choice from this group would be the wholegrain cereals, such as those found in wholemeal bread, wholemeal flour, and the wholewheat breakfast cereals, for example, Shredded Wheat, Puffed Wheat, Bran Flakes, and All Bran. It is thought that the presence of fibre in these foods reduces the rate of release of sugar into the blood after digestion, and this is much better for controlling diabetes. Those carbohydrates rich in fibre are listed in Appendix 2, page 99.

Fig. 3.5
Some common carbohydrate foods

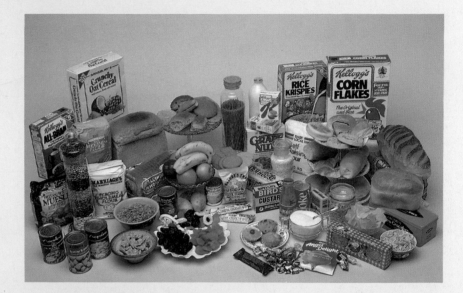

- It is important to remember that potatoes do not deserve their label as 'fattening', as an average boiled or jacket potato contains a similar amount of calories to a very small portion of meat or fish. You should, however, avoid potatoes which have had fat added to them, e.g. chipped and roast potatoes.
- You must avoid sweet and sugar foods, such as cakes, soft drinks, jams etc. (see Table 1).
- Diabetic products should also be avoided, as they are high in calories. Avoid products with the statement 'Not suitable for over-weight diabetics' on them.
- Packet and bottled sauces may be high in sugar and calories and should be avoided.

Dairy products

- This important group, which includes milk, cheese and yoghurt (Fig. 3.6), can contribute far too many calories to your daily diet and should be carefully controlled.

- Milk is a useful food to include every day, but half a pint is sufficient. If larger quantities are needed, fresh, skimmed or semi-skimmed milk can be used.

- Cheese is high in calories and should only be taken as the main portion of a meal, in place of meat, fish or poultry. The amount to have at any one time is about the size of a small matchbox. If preferred, a more generous helping of cottage cheese or reduced-fat soft cheese can be taken instead.

- Yoghurt is a popular dairy product and can be included in a weight-reducing diet, but it is better to buy plain, unsweetened or reduced-calorie yoghurt and add a small helping of fruit, rather than to use sweetened fruit yoghurt which is much higher in calories and often less filling.

- Other milk products, such as evaporated milk, can be taken in small quantities, but sweetened dairy products, for instance condensed milk, must be avoided.

Fig. 3.6
Dairy products should be eaten with caution.

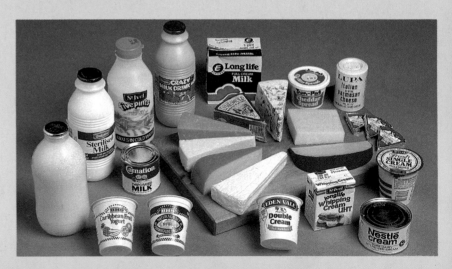

Protein foods

- This group includes meat, fish, poultry and eggs, all of which contain a large number of calories (see Appendix 2). It is usually sufficient to have one or two small helpings from this group each day (Fig. 3.7).

- Ensure that all fat is trimmed from the meat, and that fat or oil is skimmed from the cooked dishes whenever possible.

- Fish tends to be low in fat, and even the oilier fish, such as mackerel, when grilled or baked as opposed to fried, is suitable.

- Some meat products, such as sausages, paté and tinned meats contain more fat than most other meats, and therefore should not be eaten more frequently than once or twice a week.

- It is important to remember that margarine, butter, oil and lard all contain large amounts of calories and should be used very sparingly. Half a pound of butter or margarine should last at least two to three weeks. Many people find that the low-fat spreads such as Outline, Gold, Slimspread etc. are useful alternatives, but even so the amounts to be taken in any one day should still be carefully controlled.

Fig. 3.7
Protein foods.

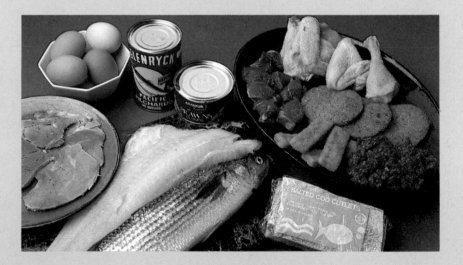

Fruit and vegetables

- This group (Fig. 3.8) forms a particularly valuable dietary constituent, because most fruit and vegetables are low calorie foods, which also have the advantage of adding bulk to the diet.

- A selection of fruit and vegetables should be included in the daily diet.

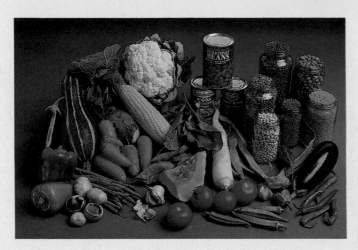

Fig. 3.8
Fruit and vegetables are essential
for a healthy diet.

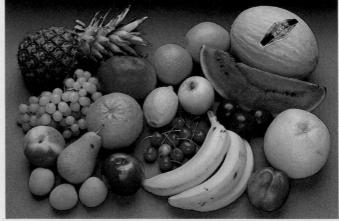

Cooking

The method of cooking is very important. Ideal cooking methods are braising, stewing, dry roasting, grilling, baking in foil, poaching and scrambling.

Frying and roasting should be avoided — for example, fried or roast potatoes are much more fattening than boiled or baked potatoes. A useful maxim is: <u>avoid the frying pan — grill instead.</u>

Useful hints when starting your diet

The first few weeks of your diet will be the most difficult to cope with. Not only will you have to plan your eating pattern carefully, but you will have to resist the temptation to eat those foods which could prove harmful. Here are some hints to help you through this difficult initial period of your diet:

● **Never miss meals**

This only makes you more hungry and therefore more likely to eat extra later on. When you diet, it is important to continue the diet long enough to show weight loss. If you diet too strictly and miss meals, you might be discouraged and give up after only a week. This would achieve nothing.

● **Reduce your portions of food**

Get used to smaller portions and fill up on the foods which you can safely eat in larger quantities, such as vegetables and salad.

● **Do not buy special slimming products**

These are unnecessary and in many cases are very expensive. It is better to learn which every-day foods you can eat.

● **Plan your diet**

Discuss your diet with the person who is cooking for you and ask them to help you by planning meals accordingly. If you are in charge of the cooking, ensure you cook the right amount of food, so there are no leftovers available for second helpings.

● **Get used to eating more slowly**

The slower you eat, the fuller you are likely to feel and the less likely you are to nibble snacks afterwards.

● **Avoid impulsive eating**

A dangerous time is when you are out shopping. Always try to have something to eat before you go out, then you will be less tempted by the rows of food you should avoid!

● Snack on the right sort of food

If you get hungry, eat an extra slice of bread or an extra piece of fruit, rather than something more concentrated, such as cake, sweets or cheese.

If you do break your diet, just once, it is not the end of the world, and you can always start again at the next meal.

● Get your family to co-operate

You are dieting to improve your health. This can also be of value to your family, so enlist their assistance in helping you with your diet. If you have the family's co-operation, you can all eat the same meals. For instance, whereas you might have served steak and kidney pudding, you can offer steak and kidney instead.

● Don't dream about food!

When you are dieting, it is easy to become obsessed by food. Try to keep your mind on other things by being busy.

● Avoid diabetic foods

Most are high in calories (see page 49).

● Be careful which sugar substitutes you use

Many are suitable, but some should be avoided (see page 49).

● Take care with alcohol

Alcohol is high in calories (see page 50).

● When eating out, select your food carefully

Avoid sweet and fatty foods (see page 51).

Summary

Dieting is never easy, but the time and effort required will, in due course, be amply rewarded. By tackling your weight problem now, you will not only help to control your diabetes, but will also probably make a significant improvement in your general health and feeling of well-being.

Now is also the time to learn which foods you should and should not eat, and the most suitable method of cooking them.

DIET IF YOUR WEIGHT IS NORMAL

Principles

Your food can be divided into three groups:

Food which should be avoided **completely**,
e.g. food containing large amounts of sugar.

Food which can be eaten with some care and regulated to
a certain extent, e.g. refined starch carbohydrate (low in
fibre) and full-fat milk and milk products, and some fats.

Food which can be eaten regularly, providing your weight
does not become excessive.

To help you identify the group to which a particular food belongs, a
colour coding system is used throughout this section. Thus, foods
to be avoided are keyed with red, yellow indicates foods to be
eaten with caution or regulated, and green identifies foods which
may be eaten regularly.

The special diet you follow should enable you to maintain your
weight without causing you to feel hungry. Such a diet will have to
be worked out with you, in the first instance, by your doctor or
dietitian, who will suggest a specific carbohydrate allowance,
but some general guidelines are given below.

Foods to be avoided

Avoid all very sweet foods and drinks, which cause a rapid rise in blood sugar.

By cutting out sweet foods you are minimizing the amount of sugar which has to be disposed of by your reduced insulin supply. A detailed list of these is given in Table 2 opposite.

Fig. 3.9
A range of common foods which, because of their high sugar content, should be avoided.

a. Sweets and chocolates have a very high sugar content, especially fruit drops and pastilles.

b. These foods rapidly affect the blood sugar. Honey is often mistakenly believed to be suitable for those with diabetes.

c. Asian and West Indian sweetmeats, which are offered as part of hospitality and at festivals, should be eaten as 'small tastes' only.

d. Sweet biscuits and cakes should be substituted with high-fibre, low-sugar alternatives.

e. Instant desserts and sweetened cereals should be replaced with unsweetened alternatives.

f. These highly sweetened drinks should be avoided.

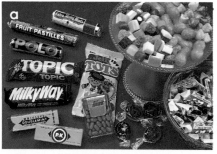

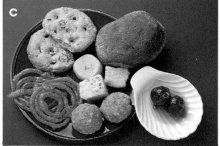

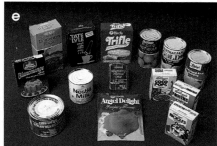

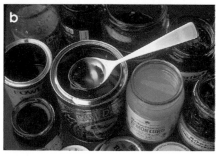

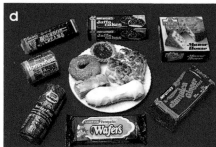

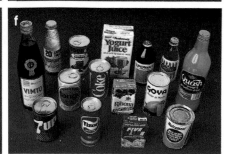

TABLE 2 Foods to be avoided

The foods listed below are high in sugar and have virtually no nutritional value:

Marmalade */jam */honey *

Mincemeat/lemon curd

Golden syrup

Black treacle

Sugar

Glucose

Glucose tablets

Fizzy and mixer drinks *, cordials * and squashes *, unless marked 'no sugar'/'low calorie'.

Minerals *

Coca-Cola *

Lemonade *

Tonic *, ginger ale *, bitter lemon * etc.

Bottled sauces and chutneys (in large amounts)

Buns

Pastries

Sweet biscuits

Sweets and chocolates

Fruit tinned in syrup *

*Low-sugar alternatives are available.

For further information refer to 'Countdown', published by the British Diabetic Association.

Fig. 3.10
Some examples of foods containing
10g (1 'exchange') of carbohydrate.

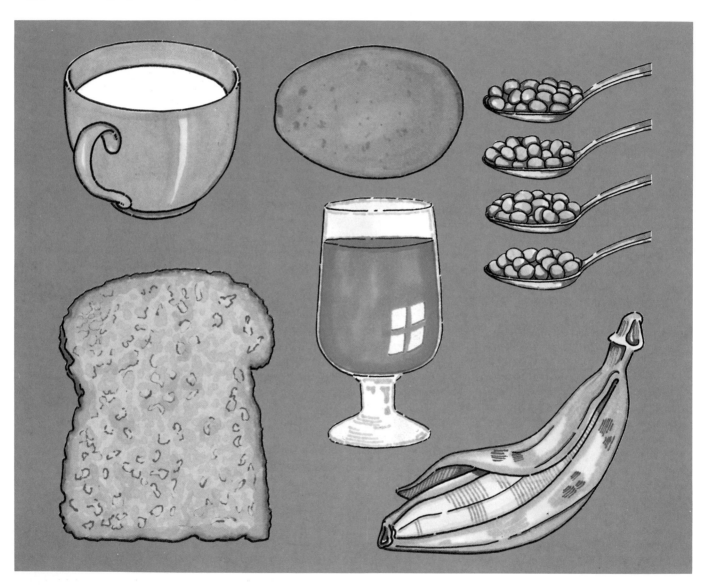

Foods to be eaten with care and in regulated amounts

Carbohydrates

How much carbohydrate?

The first point to remember is that your diet must contain enough carbohydrate to ensure a reasonable level of blood sugar, in order to provide the fuel your body needs. You **CANNOT** cut out all foods providing sugar. This would merely induce your body to make more sugar from its reserves, thereby causing you to lose weight and become unwell. Starvation is no treatment for any type of diabetes.

The total amount of carbohydrate you need will be determined for you. Usually almost half your total energy (calorie) requirement is supplied by carbohydrates. This will be subdivided so that you take most of it at main meals and smaller amounts at snack times. To help you control your carbohydrate intake, and still enjoy a varied and interesting diet, a system of 'exchanges' (also called 'portions', 'rations', or 'lines') is used. If you look at Table 3, page 40, carbohydrates have been listed in single household measures, i.e. tablespoons, cups, slices etc, so that each measure of whichever type of food you prefer contains 10 g of carbohydrate, called a 'portion' or an 'exchange'. All of these are equivalent (Fig. 3.10). Thus, one Weetabix is equivalent to one thin slice of bread, one egg-sized potato or two tablespoons of flour. A more detailed list is given in Appendix 2, page 99.

If it has been decided that you need five portions for each main meal, you can then simply select those you prefer, e.g. two portions of bread, two of cereal and one of fruit, or any other mixture. Your snacks can be similarly varied. In these calculations you should not forget additions, such as milk with cereal.

It is not necessary to weigh food. With the help of lists and advice from your dietitian, you should not find difficulty in basing your quantities on household measures.

TABLE 3 Carbohydrate exchanges [†]

Foods in this list contain carbohydrate (starch) in substantial amounts.

These foods are listed in exchanges, which are equal in carbohydrate value, so you may 'exchange' any of these for another on your daily menu.

Each exchange = 10g of carbohydrate

High-fibre foods are marked: *good fibre content

**very good fibre content

Spoon measures are standard kitchen spoons.

Bread and biscuits
* 1 small slice of wholemeal bread [††]
* ½ large thick slice of bread [††]
* 1 small roll [††]
2 crispbreads
* 1 digestive or wholemeal biscuit
2 cream crackers or water biscuits
2 plain or semi-sweet biscuits

Cereals
** 2 level tablespoons wholemeal flour
1½ level tablespoons white flour
** 3 level tablespoons uncooked porridge
4 tablespoons wholemeal breakfast cereal, e.g. **Branflakes
** 12 Shreddies
** 1 Weetabix or ⅔ Shredded Wheat
2 tablespoons cooked pasta, e.g. macaroni
2 level tablespoons cooked rice
1 level tablespoon custard powder
2 level teaspoons sago/tapioca/semolina
Choose wholemeal bread, wholewheat pasta or brown rice where possible, as they are rich in fibre.

Vegetables

**4 level tablespoons baked beans
**2 level tablespoons lentils (before cooking)
**4 level tablespoons tinned or well cooked 'dried' beans
2 small beetroot
1 small parsnip
1 egg-sized potato (boiled, roast)
1 scoop mashed potato
*1 small jacket potato
**½ medium corn-on-the-cob
**5 tablespoons sweetcorn

Fruit

1 apple, 1 orange, 1 pear, 1 peach, 1 small banana, 10 grapes, 12 cherries, 2 dessert plums, **2 large prunes, 1 slice pineapple, 15 strawberries, 2 tangerines
*2 level tablespoons currants, raisins or sultanas
1 small bowl stewed fruit
1 small glass (4 fluid oz) fruit juice, (e.g. apple, grapefruit, orange, pineapple)
4-6 chestnuts

Milk

1 cup (⅓ pint) whole or skimmed milk
1 carton (small) plain yoghurt or ½ carton fruit yoghurt
6 tablespoons (3 fluid oz) evaporated milk

Miscellaneous

Use these only occasionally to make up your exchanges, as they contain a lot of fat, a lot of sugar, or are low in fibre.

1 cup of soup (tinned or packet)	2 sausages
2 level teaspoons Horlicks, Ovaltine	4 large chips
2 bun-size batter puddings	
1 small brickette (or scoop) ice cream	

† More detailed lists are available in Appendix 2, page 99.
†† Sliced bread varies according to the brand; the carbohydrate content will be found on the packaging. For further details of the carbohydrate content of these and other manufactured foods, you should refer to 'Countdown', published by the British Diabetic Association.

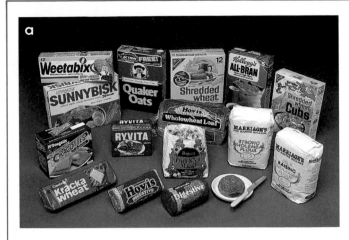

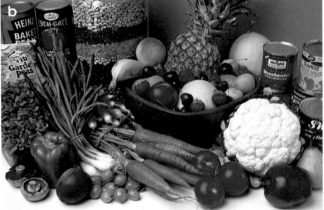

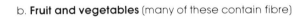

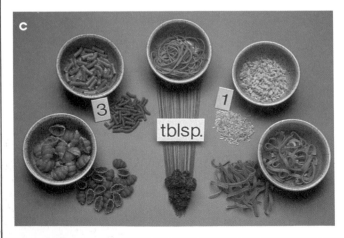

Fig. 3.11
The best choice of carbohydrate foods.

a. **Fibre-containing foods**

b. **Fruit and vegetables** (many of these contain fibre)

c. **Pasta and wholegrain rice**

The best choice of carbohydrates

● **Fibre** reduces the rate of release of sugar into the blood after digestion, and this, of course, is much better for diabetic control. Carbohydrates rich in fibre include the wholegrain cereals, such as those found in wholemeal bread, wholemeal flour, and whole wheat breakfast cereals, for example Shredded Wheat, Puffed Wheat, Bran Flakes and All Bran (Fig. 3.11).

You should select from Table 3 (see also Appendix 2) those carbohydrates with a high fibre content. These should provide up to two thirds of your total carbohydrate requirements.

● **Fruit and vegetables** should always be included in the daily diet. Those that contain carbohydrate should be included in your total daily intake, as indicated in Table 3, some can be eaten in unlimited quantities (see page 46) and many are high in fibre.

Dairy Products

● **Milk** (Fig. 3.12) is a useful food to include every day, but does contain sugar (see Table 3) and must be considered as an exchange or portion.

Fig. 3.12
Dairy products should be eaten in regulated amounts.

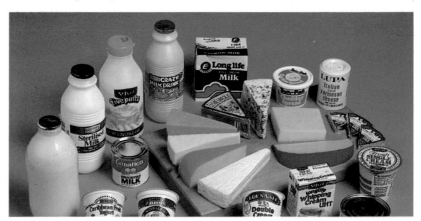

- **Yoghurt** is a popular dairy product, but it is better to buy a reduced-sugar yoghurt, or a plain, unsweetened yoghurt and add a small helping of fruit, rather than normal sweetened fruit yoghurt which contains a lot of sugar.
- **Other milk products,** such as evaporated milk, can be taken in small quantities, but sweetened dairy products, for instance condensed milk, must be avoided.

Be extra careful with these foods

- **Fats** (Fig. 3.13a and b) should be eaten with some restraint. They are a concentrated form of calories, which easily lead to overweight, and in excess may cause other health problems.
- **Meat products** (Fig. 3.13a) which are particularly high in fat, such as sausages and meat pies, should be eaten in limited amounts. Also, you should remove the fat from the meat.
- **Cheese, cream, butter and margarine** should be limited. Do not nibble fatty foods.
  Spread butter and other spreads sparingly.
  Try replacing milk with skimmed or semi-skimmed milk.

If you feel hungry and you are not overweight, it is likely that you need more carbohydrate. It is not wise to base every meal on a large portion of meat, fish or cheese. If you are in doubt about your allowance, ask the advice of your doctor or dietitian.

Ideal cooking methods are braising, stewing, dry roasting, grilling, baking in foil, poaching or scrambling. A useful maxim is: avoid the frying pan — grill instead.

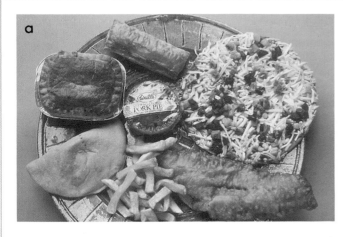

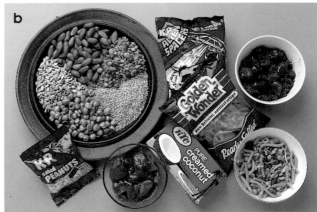

Fig. 3.13
Extra care is required when eating these foods.

a. Many popular foods contain a high level of 'hidden' fat, particularly meat products, pastry and fried food such as fish and chips.

b. Other foods with a high 'hidden' fat content, include natural foods, such as nuts and seeds, and processed foods, such as crisps.

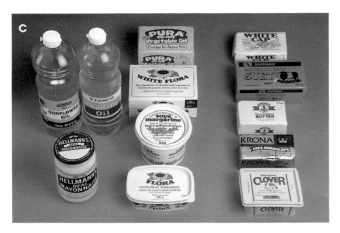

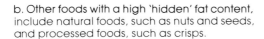

c. All of these 'visible' fats should be limited. Full-fat milk, as used in some yoghurts, and evaporated milk are best reduced.

Foods which can be eaten regularly

Fruits and vegetables

Some fruits and most vegetables contain negligible amounts of carbohydrate, are low in calories, and can be eaten in generous quantities. Examples are listed in Table 4, opposite.

Proteins — lean meat, poultry, fish and eggs

- To have pleasant and nutritional meals, the balance of energy or calories is provided by protein (and fat). As Westerners, we eat considerably more protein than we really need.
- Providing you take care to avoid a very fat diet, lean meat, poultry, fish and eggs (Fig. 3.14a) can be eaten as normal.

Beverages

Drinks listed in Table 4, do not contain sugar. Soft drinks, listed in Table 2, should be avoided, as they contain a lot of sugar. It should be remembered that drinks taken with milk, such as tea and cocoa, contain both calories and carbohydrate.

Fig. 3.14
Foods which can be eaten regularly.

a. **Protein-containing foods** — care should be taken to limit the intake of fat.

b. **Beverages** — sugar-free mixer drinks may be drunk freely.

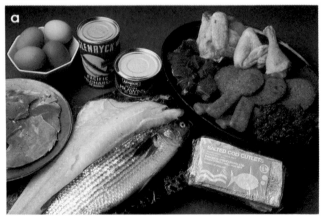
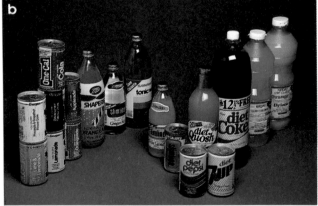

TABLE 4 Foods which can be eaten freely

Vegetables

Cauliflower	Marrow	Tomatoes
Runner beans	Mushrooms	Peppers
Carrots	Celery	Swede
Peas	Onions	Turnip

All green leafy vegetables
Frozen and fresh peas
Salad vegetables

Fruit

Cranberries	Lemons	Rhubarb
Gooseberries	Loganberries	Redcurrants
½ Grapefruit		

Beverages

Tea	Bovril	Tomato juice
Coffee	Marmite	Lemon juice
Oxo	Soda water	Clear soups

Sugar-free squashes and 'mixers'

Seasonings

Pepper	Pickles	Spices
Mustard	Herbs	Stock cubes
Vinegar	Essences and food colourings	

Sweetening agents

Only tablet and liquid saccharine sweetener, aspartame and acesulfame-K.

Your family's diet

Although the type of diet outlined above is designed for the specific needs of a person with diabetes, it is a particularly healthy diet in so far as it is based on a minimal sugar and fat intake, and an increase in the consumption of fruit, vegetables and fibre-containing foods. Consequently, it is recommended that the whole family should be offered the benefits of meals based on this type of diet.

Fig. 3.15
Food for people with diabetes can be enjoyed by the whole family. Such food is not only healthier, but can be just as tasty as more conventional dishes.

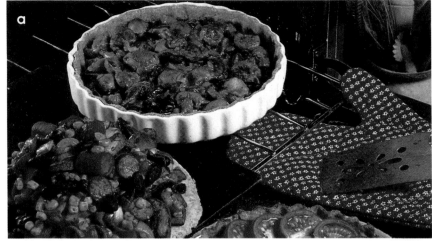

a. Frankfurter pizza, Mixed grill flan and Tuna flan.

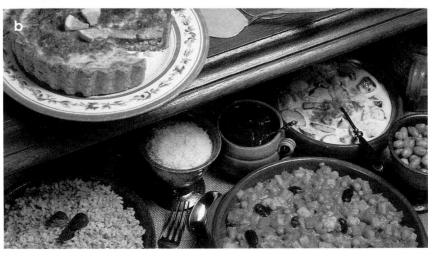

b. Cottage cheese quiche and Vegetable curry.

Eating out

As your knowledge about your diet increases, you will gain more confidence about eating out, and will be able to select from the menus those foods which are most appropriate. For those of normal weight, eating out need not be restricted.

Fig. 3.16
Eating out.
With a little extra care you can eat out and still follow your diet.

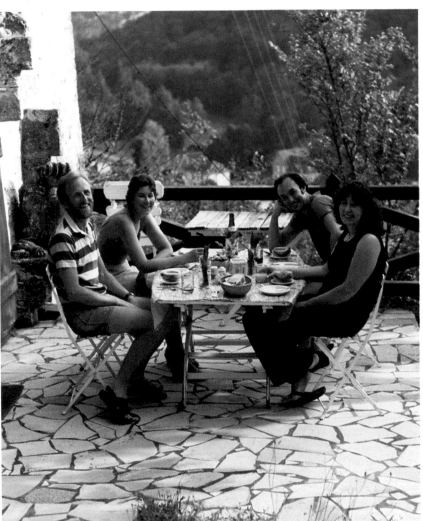

If you are at all concerned about the suitability of certain foods in a restaurant, do not be afraid to ask.

Wherever possible:

- Select generous portions of vegetables

- Cut down on fats and sugar

- Choose baked, grilled or boiled food, as opposed to fried or roasted.

However, an occasional indiscretion, although it may lead to a temporary rise in blood sugar, will not do any long-term harm.

Of course, eating with friends or relatives should pose no problems. If you let them know the foods you would prefer not to eat, any embarrassment will be readily avoided.

If you need help

If you should have any problems with your diet, do not be afraid to ask for help from your doctor or dietitian. Very good guidance can be obtained from the many diabetic cookery books and from the extensive lists of foods now available, such as 'Countdown', published by the British Diabetic Association.

Summary

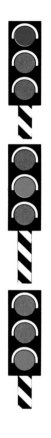

Your food can be divided into three groups:

> **Food which should be avoided completely, e.g. food containing large amounts of sugar.**

> **Food which can be eaten with some care and regulated to a certain extent, e.g. refined starch carbohydrate (low in fibre) and full-fat milk and milk products, and some fats.**

> **Food which can be eaten regularly, providing your weight does not become excessive.**

Planning your diet consists of the following steps:

- Determining the total number of carbohydrate portions per day

- Deciding when to have the portions

- Selecting the type of food suited to your taste

- Balancing meals and snacks with foods freely allowed, avoiding those containing sugar.

'Diabetic' foods

These foods are usually sweet, as cane sugar has been substituted with other sweeteners. They are best avoided, not only because they are very expensive, but because they are very often high in calories, and therefore fattening. Some specialist products, however, may add variety to the diet. These include the wide range of sugar-free drinks, fruits tinned in natural juices, reduced-sugar preserves, and sugar-free sweets and chewing gum (Fig. 3.17).

Fig. 3.17
Special 'diabetic' foods.
Sugar-free and low-sugar drinks are suitable for those with diabetes.

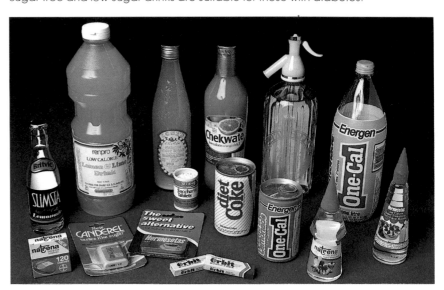

Sugar substitutes — which ones?

Saccharine, saccharine-based sweeteners, acesulfame K or aspartame can be used by any one with diabetes. Examples of these are the various tablet and liquid sweeteners, such as Hermesetas, Sweetex, Saxin, Natrena, Canderel, etc. (Fig. 3.17). Powder sweeteners, which are mixtures of saccharine and sugar, or saccharine and milk sugar, or saccharine and sorbitol, or fructose (fruit sugar) should not be used without individual advice from your dietitian, but they may be useful in baking or preserve making.

Alcohol

Alcohol need not be avoided, but some care should be exercised.

- Alcohol is a source of a considerable number of calories, which can cause significant weight problems (if you are overweight you should take advice from your doctor).
- Most beers, lagers and ciders are high in carbohydrate and calories. Normally, if you are on a weight-reducing diet, a maximum of one drink per day would be permitted as part of the calorie allowance. It is inadvisable to drink more than an average of three drinks daily on a regular basis and less is preferable.
- Particular care should be taken with beers described as 'low in carbohydrate'. They are not only expensive but have a higher alcohol and calories content than ordinary beers.
- Mixers which contain sugar should be avoided completely (see Table 2). Use 'slimline' varieties.
- Sweet wines are very variable in sugar content and are best avoided.
- Avoid liqueurs.
- Home-made wines and beers are very variable in both sugar and alcohol content.

Remember:

- **Never drink on an empty stomach**
- **Drink moderate quantities only**
- **Never drink and drive.**

TABLET TREATMENT

When to use tablets

When diet alone is not fully successful, then there may be loss of control of your diabetes. In such circumstances tablets may be given in combination with the special diet — tablet treatment is never employed by itself.

Which tablets to use?

Two types of tablets are commonly used to treat non-insulin dependent diabetes, the commoner being those that work by stimulating your pancreas to produce more insulin. These are listed in Table 5.

Occasionally, however, these tablets alone are not completely effective, and in such cases an additional tablet, called metformin (trade name, Glucophage), may also be prescribed. Sometimes metformin may be used on its own.

Remember, too, that you must stick to your diet when taking tablets. You cannot expect the tablets to control your sugar level if you eat what you like — they are not a substitute for diet!

TABLE 5 Tablets used to treat diabetes

Chemical name	Brand name	Chemical name	Brand name
SULPHONYLUREA TYPE			
Acetohexamide	Dimelor	Gliclazide	Diamicron
Chlorpropamide	Diabinese	Glipizide	Glibenese
	Glymese		Minodiab
	Melitase	Gliquidone	Glurenorm
Glibenclamide	Daonil	Glymidine	Gondafon
	Semi-daonil	Tolazamide	Tolanase
	Euglucon	Tolbutamide	Glyconon
	Libanil		Pramidex
	Malix		Rastinon
Glibornuride	Glutril		
BIGUANIDE TYPE			
Metformin	Glucophage		

Some important questions about tablet treatment

Are you at risk until your blood sugar returns to normal?

Initially, your treatment with diet alone, or with a combination of diet and tablets, will take a few weeks to return your blood sugar to a normal level. During this delay, however, you will come to no harm, because the long-term complications of diabetes, which affect the eyes, kidneys and nerves, take many years to develop.

What happens if the tablets do not work?

If your blood sugar remains high, in spite of taking tablets — even perhaps after the addition of metformin — and you are carefully following your diet, your doctor may recommend insulin. In the majority of people, however, this is never necessary. Most instances where diabetes is not brought under control, or where control is not maintained, are due to a failure to follow the diet.

Is there a risk of going into a diabetic coma?

No, this is very rare in your type of diabetes. It never occurs when you are well. If you should become sick, vomit, lose your appetite and become very thirsty and your tests (see Chapter 4, page 59) are positive, you should consult your doctor in order to avoid unnecessary risks.

Can tablets cause side effects?

Side effects are rare. The sulphonylurea tablets cause no ill effects in the many thousands of people who take them. Skin rashes may occur very occasionally. Also, slight swelling of the ankles may be noted in the early stages of treatment, and weight gain of a few pounds can occur.

Some people react with mild stomach discomfort to metformin.

If you are taking chlorpropamide tablets you may develop flushing of the face after drinking alcohol. Although discomforting, it is quite harmless and lasts only a few minutes before disappearing. There is no need to stop drinking alcohol, but if the problem becomes troublesome, a change of tablet might be considered.

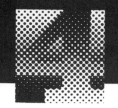

Is your treatment effective?

It is clear from the last chapter that the aim of treatment is to return your blood sugar to normal and to maintain it at that level. Unfortunately, how you feel is not a reliable guide to the level of your blood sugar, and symptoms such as thirst, weight loss and passing large amounts of urine appear only if the diabetes is badly out of control. Even with moderately high levels of blood sugar — the sort of levels which can, over a period of years, lead to serious complications — you may have no symptoms. Clearly, some form of test is required which can be repeated at frequent intervals, in order to ensure that your control is being maintained at an acceptable level.

Blood tests v. urine tests

Blood sugar levels can be assessed either directly by means of blood tests, or indirectly by urine tests. Home blood tests are usually unnecessary for those with diabetes not requiring insulin. Urine tests have the important advantage that they are painless. Also, because they are much simpler to perform, they can be carried out easily at home. Therefore for the majority of those with non-insulin dependent diabetes, regular urine testing will provide an effective guide to blood sugar levels.

Urine tests

How urine tests work and their interpretation

When the blood sugar rises, a point is reached at which it starts to leak into the urine. In the majority this will happen whenever the blood sugar is too high, usually above about 10 mmol/l. Therefore, if the blood sugar has exceeded this threshold level since you last passed urine, a test for sugar in the urine will be positive (Fig. 4.1a). If the blood sugar is below this level (normal), the urine tests will be negative (Fig. 4.1b). Therefore, all urine tests, should be negative with your type of diabetes.

Fig. 4.1
How urine tests work.

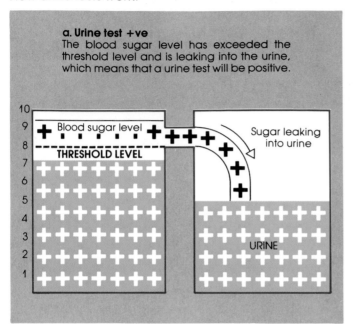

a. Urine test +ve
The blood sugar level has exceeded the threshold level and is leaking into the urine, which means that a urine test will be positive.

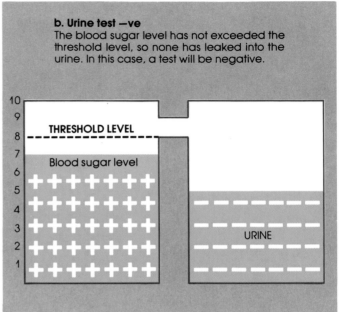

b. Urine test —ve
The blood sugar level has not exceeded the threshold level, so none has leaked into the urine. In this case, a test will be negative.

How often should you test?

To start with, you will be asked to test several times a day, because this will help you to understand what causes the blood sugar to rise. As your urine tests become negative, i.e. as your blood sugar returns to normal, two or three tests a week may be all that are required to reassure you that all remains well.

Stress and illness also increase your blood sugar. Therefore, you would be wise to test your urine several times a day during any illness — even a cold or 'flu' — in order to discover whether your treatment needs to be modified.

When should you test?

Clearly, once treatment has begun to take effect, you will only wish to know if at any time the blood sugar is abnormally high. Therefore,

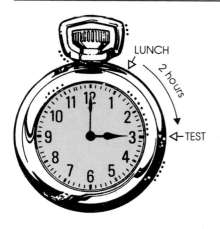

LUNCH

2 hours

TEST

Fig. 4.2
Keep a record of your urine test results.

perform your urine test two hours after a main meal, since it is at this time that your blood sugar will be at its highest.

Keep a record of your tests

Isolated tests of the urine are of little value, but a regular record (Fig. 4.2) gives a much better idea of the level of control being achieved. Such a record will be of particular value when you attend your doctor or clinic for your regular medical check-up. Each test should be recorded on a chart or in a book.

Date / Time		Urine Glucose				Remarks:
		8am	2.30 pm	6pm	10pm	
Mon		nil				
Tue		nil				
Wed			++			After meal
Thur		nil				
Fri					nil	
Sat						
Sun		+++				Heavy meal night before

Which urine tests?

Three tests (Fig. 4.3) are commonly available in the United Kingdom:

● **Clinitest,** which involves adding a tablet to urine diluted with water in a test tube, and observing the change in colour.

● **Diastix,** which involves placing a strip of special paper in the stream of urine, and observing the colour change.

● **Diabur-test 5000,** used similarly to Diastix.

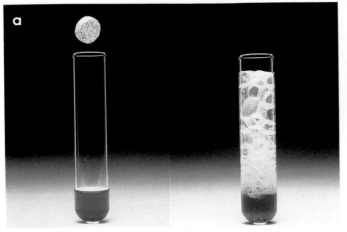

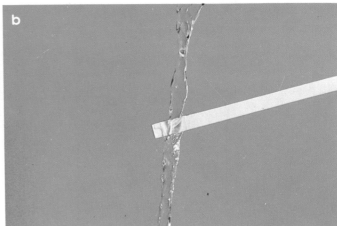

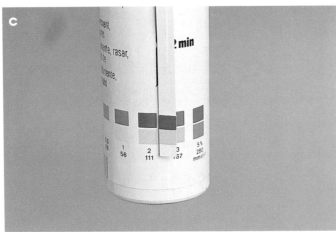

Fig. 4.3
Urine test kits.
a. Clinitest
b. Diastix
c. Diabur-Test 5000

All tests are quite satisfactory. Clinitest is easier to observe, but has the disadvantage of requiring you to collect a sample of urine to put into a tube for testing. Diastix and Diabur-Test 5000, on the other hand, are rather simpler to use, but if your sight is not perfect, may be less accurate.

You will, of course, be shown how to test your urine when you first develop diabetes, but if you have any doubts as to whether you are doing it correctly, check with your doctor or clinic. For reference purposes, full details of the three common tests are provided in Appendix 1, page 91. Remember that urine tests depend on a colour change, so if you cannot see well, or you are colour blind, you may not be able to detect the change and the tests may need to be done for you.

Blood tests

When are blood tests performed?

Blood tests will be carried out when you attend the clinic or visit your doctor, in order to check that your urine tests are providing reliable information about your actual blood picture.

Although you may feel unhappy about handling urine, it is, in most people, perfectly sterile and clean. However, the techniques now available for home blood sugar tests make it possible for you to avoid urine tests if you so wish. Such blood tests require only a single drop of blood, which you can obtain by pricking your finger. It should be stressed, though, that most people with non-insulin dependent diabetes do not need to perform direct measurements of their blood sugar routinely.

Regular weighing

Regular weighing is helpful in assessing control. Your weight should not exceed the average weight for your height. Obesity aggravates the long-term effects of diabetes, so if you are overweight you must get your weight down to normal and keep it there.

Factors leading to loss of control

In certain circumstances diabetes may go out of control unexpectedly. The 5 most common causes of loss of control are:

1. **The development of an acute infection**
   - Urinary infection
   - Large boils, carbuncles or abscesses
   - Severe chest infection
   - More seriously — gastroenteritis associated with vomiting.

2. **After starting certain medications**
   - Especially with steroids (prednisone, cortisone)
   - Sometimes with certain water tablets (diuretics) used in the treatment of blood pressure and heart disease
   - Some tablets and medicines, especially cough syrup, contain a lot of sugar and should be avoided.

3. Stressful situations

When people with diabetes are worried or anxious, they may find that their diabetes becomes more difficult to control.

4. Failure to respond to tablets

In some people with diabetes, the tablets may lose their effect after a period of satisfactory control. Changing to a different tablet may correct the situation, but a few people may need to be re-stabilized with insulin.

5. Failure to follow the advised treatment

Those with diabetes who abandon their diet, stop taking their tablets, or both, will almost certainly become badly controlled, although the deterioration may be quite a gradual process.

In any of these situations, the blood sugar may rise and large amounts of sugar may be passed in the urine. Most illnesses, such as 'flu' and colds, are of short duration and have no significant long-term effects, though the blood sugar, and hence urine tests, may show increases for a day or so. An occasional dietary indiscretion may also show itself in a similar way. If, however, the urine tests become positive for sugar for more than a couple of days, you may need additional treatment and you should contact your doctor.

Vomiting and severe diarrhoea are, however, of greater significance, because they may cause the loss of a substantial amount of fluid and consequently an increased thirst. Although a person with non-insulin dependent diabetes does not develop keto-acidosis (diabetic coma), the salt balance in the blood may become disturbed. If, having taken adequate fluid by mouth, you feel very thirsty and all your tests are positive, you must consult your general practitioner. Very rarely, he may decide you need admission to hospital, so that the large quantity of fluid you have lost can be replaced by intravenous drip, and also because insulin may be required, at least temporarily.

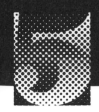

The long-term effects of diabetes and your general health

Treatment of diabetes very rapidly restores health to normal; the symptoms disappear quite quickly, and weight and energy return to normal.

However, after many years of diabetes, some of the body's tissues may be damaged. The eyes, kidneys, and some nerves, mainly those to the feet, are most susceptible. These problems, however, are likely to develop only after many years of poor blood sugar control, and thus occur most frequently in those who pay least attention to their diabetes. Many people with diabetes are completely spared these problems, and even after more than forty years of diabetes, show no trace of any complications.

Foot problems

These are rather more common in your type of diabetes, but can usually be prevented with care. Therefore, this section is particularly important to you.

Damage to the feet

Long-term diabetes sometimes results in nerve damage (called neuritis or neuropathy), which mainly affects the feeling in the feet. The hazard of this condition is that the majority of those in whom it occurs are not aware of the subtle decrease of sensation in their feet.

The feet normally undergo a lot of wear and tear, and any injuries are usually noticed because of discomfort. If, however, discomfort is not felt because of neuritis, increasing damage to the feet may pass unnoticed. In addition, these injuries may be further aggravated by diminished circulation. Ulceration and infection which then occur, can be very serious and result in prolonged periods off work, in bed, or in hospital, and sometimes require operations or even amputations. To a large extent these injuries can, however, be avoided, if proper care is taken of the feet.

Therefore, the 'do's' and 'don'ts' of foot care are of great importance, and you should read the following section carefully.

Prevention of foot problems

Scrupulous attention to care of the feet can prevent serious complications. The following measures and precautions are **ESSENTIAL** for **ALL** those with diabetes.

Inspecting your feet

● Inspect your feet regularly — ideally, daily — and if you cannot do this yourself, ask a friend to do it for you. This inspection is important because you may not always be able to feel bruises or sores.

● Seek advice if you develop any cracks or breaks in the skin, any calluses or corns, or your feet are swollen or throbbing. Advice from a State Registered Chiropodist is freely available under the National Health Service.

Washing your feet

● Wash your feet daily in warm water.

● Use a mild type of toilet soap.

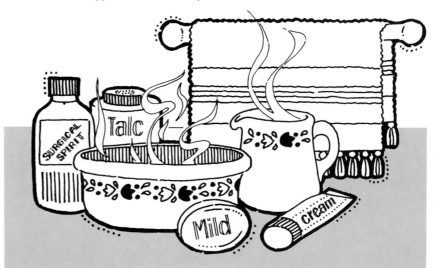

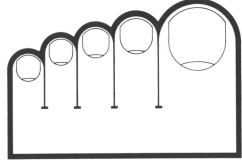

- Rinse the skin well after washing. Dry your feet carefully, blotting between the toes with a soft towel.
- Dust with plain talc, wiping off any excess and ensuring that it does not clog between the toes.
- If your skin is too dry, sparingly apply a little cream containing lanolin, or an emulsifying ointment. This should be gently rubbed in after bathing the feet.
- If your skin is too moist, wipe your feet with surgical spirit, especially between the toes. When the spirit has dried, dust the skin with talcum powder or baby powder.

Nail cutting

- When your toenails need cutting, do this after bathing, when the nails are soft and pliable. Do not cut them too short.
- Never cut the corners of your nails too far back at the sides, but allow the cut to follow the natural line of the end of the toe.
- Never use a sharp instrument to clean under your nails or in the nail grooves at the sides of the nails.
- If your toe nails are painful, or if you experience difficulty in cutting them, consult your chiropodist.

Heat and cold

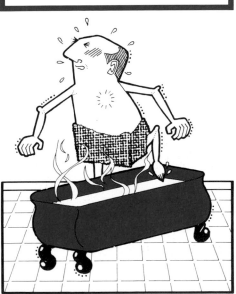

- Be careful to avoid baths which are too hot.
- Do not sit too close to heaters or fires, and protect your legs and feet by covering them with a rug.
- Before getting into bed, remove hot water bottles, unless they are fabric covered. Electric under-blankets should be switched off or unplugged.
- Do not allow wet feet to get cold. Even if they do not feel cold, dry them quickly and put on dry socks, in order to maintain body warmth.
- Do not use hot fomentations or poultices.

Shoes

Shoes must fit properly and provide adequate support. In fact, careful fitting and choice of shoes is probably the most important

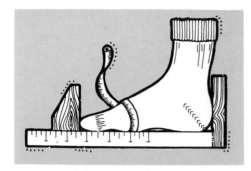

measure you can take to prevent foot problems. Therefore:

- Wear comfortable, good-fitting shoes with soft uppers. Lace-ups with medium heels are ideal.
- Never accept shoes that you feel must be 'broken in'.
- When buying new shoes, always try them on, and rely on the advice of a qualified shoe fitter. Shoes must always be the correct shape for your feet.
- Slippers do not provide adequate support. Therefore, they should be worn only for short periods, and not throughout the day. Do not walk about in bare feet.
- Do not wear garters.

Daily rule: Feel inside your shoes, before putting them on. This is important, because you may not feel nails or pieces of grit under your feet, as a result of lost sensitivity in your feet.

Corns and calluses

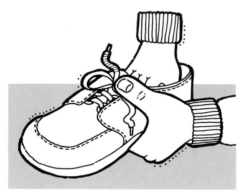

- Do not cut your corns and calluses yourself, or let a well-meaning friend cut them for you.
- Do not use corn paints or corn plasters. They contain acids which can be extremely dangerous to those with diabetes.
- Any corns, calluses, in-growing nails and other foot ailments, should be treated by a State-Registered Chiropodist.

First aid measures

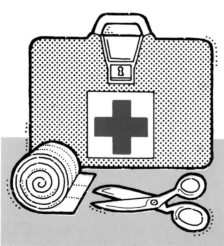

- Minor injuries, such as cuts and abrasions, can be self-treated quite adequately, by gently cleaning the area with soap and water and covering it with a sterile dressing.
- If blisters occur, do not prick them. If they burst, dress them as for a minor cut.
- Never use strong medicaments, such as iodine, Dettol, Germoline or other powerful antiseptics.
- Never place adhesive strapping directly over a wound.
- If you are in the slightest doubt about how to deal with any wound, discolouration, corns, and especially ulcers, consult your doctor.

Damage to the eyes

Two parts of the eye are affected by diabetes:

1. **The lens**

   Opacities in the lens (cataracts) are common in elderly people, and sometimes cause deterioration of vision. Cataracts occur more often in people with diabetes than in normal individuals.

2. **The retina**

   This is the sensitive part of the back of the eye, which is responsible for transmitting visual images to the brain. Diabetes quite often causes minor abnormalities of the retina, without causing deterioration of vision — a condition described by the term 'diabetic retinopathy'. However, in a minority of sufferers, vision deteriorates, and the affected eye becomes blind, usually from bleeding (haemorrhage) within the eye.

Prevention and treatment of eye damage

When cataracts seriously interfere with vision, they may be treated by surgery.

Fortunately, damage to the retina can now be treated and blindness prevented in many instances. Treatment is by laser, a process which involves aiming a fine beam of very bright light at the diseased blood vessels. It is very simple to perform and is often successful, but it has to be undertaken before sight has deteriorated too seriously.

Therefore, it is essential that you should have your eyes tested and the backs of your eyes examined regularly — ideally, annually. This can be done by an optician, by doctors in the clinic, or by an eye specialist.

Some blurring of vision may occur in the first few weeks of treatment, but this is of no consequence and nearly always resolves within a week or two — so don't get your glasses changed. Subsequently, if you should notice a sudden loss of vision in either eye, you must report to your doctor immediately.

Damage to the kidneys

Damage to the kidneys occurs less frequently than eye damage. Kidney damage must be present for many years before function begins to deteriorate, and even then a few more years usually elapse before the situation becomes serious. Unfortunately, there are no symptoms relating to kidney disease until it is quite advanced. Therefore, regular checks by your doctor are an important means of ensuring early detection of disease.

Painful neuritis

Rarely, neuritis causes pain, usually in the feet and legs, which is particularly disagreeable. A burning sensation, a feeling of pins-and-needles, with an excruciating discomfort on contact with clothes or bedclothes, are the main characteristics of this condition. Unpleasant though these symptoms are, they usually disappear in time, although it may take many months for them to do so. Very good control is an essential part of treatment, and this often requires the use of insulin. Various tablets, including pain-killers, are also used in treating this condition.

Impotence

Sometimes, nerve damage causes impotence. It should be remembered, however, that impotence is also common in those without diabetes. It is often due to psychological causes, and for this reason it is sometimes difficult to discover whether or not it is due to nerve damage resulting from diabetes.

Proper diagnosis is important, and specialist advice should be sought.

Arterial disease

Hardening and narrowing of the arteries are normal consequences of ageing, but with diabetes there may be slight acceleration of this process. Arterial disease can result in heart attacks and cause poor circulation in the feet and legs.

Treatment for these disorders is exactly the same as in those without diabetes. You should take the following precautions:
- Do not smoke
- Do not become overweight

H.M. Govt. Health Depts.' WARNING:
CIGARETTES CAN
SERIOUSLY DAMAGE YOUR HEALTH

- Have your blood pressure checked annually and treated if necessary
- Reduce the amount of fat in your diet
- Take as much exercise as you can and you will keep the risk of arterial disease to a minimum.

Associated illnesses

Very occasionally, diabetes may be associated with another illness, or it may actually be part of an illness. Sometimes, diabetes develops as a result of the treatment given for other illnesses, such as disorders of the liver and pancreas, excess iron stores in the blood, and hormonal problems involving the thyroid and adrenal glands. Generally, such problems will be identified when you first see your doctor, and treatment will be prescribed in parallel with the treatment for your diabetes.

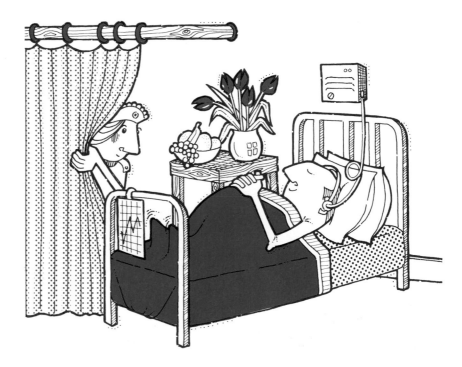

Regular medical check-ups

In the period after your diabetes has been diagnosed, your doctor may wish to see you every few weeks, until he is sure that the treatment is effective. However, when your blood sugar has been brought under control, he may want to see you perhaps every few months or, if you are very well controlled, yearly.

With your urine test records you will be able to keep a routine check on the effectiveness of your treatment. Nonetheless, from time to time it is essential that you visit your doctor or clinic, so that your treatment can be monitored, and any specific problems you might have can be dealt with.

For example:

● Your doctor will want to be sure that your tests are satisfactory. If the record of your tests shows erratic or high sugar levels, he will decide whether additional treatment is necessary.

● He will want to perform a blood test to check your control, because sometimes the urine tests may be misleading.

● He will want to ensure that you understand and are happy with the advice you have been given. This is the time for you to ask questions!

● From time to time, he will want to check whether any long-term complications have developed. It is important that these should be detected before you notice anything wrong, so that early treatment can be commenced.

● Finally, such visits provide you with an opportunity to discuss problems with, for example, your dietitian, as well as reporting any new symptoms, such as difficulty with vision or problems with your feet.

If you are not feeling well, your treatment appears not to be working, or you develop any unusual symptoms, such as worsening eyesight, or abnormal tingling in the hands or feet, report to your doctor at once — **DO NOT WAIT FOR YOUR NEXT APPOINTMENT.**

Fig. 5.1
Regular visits to your clinic are essential.

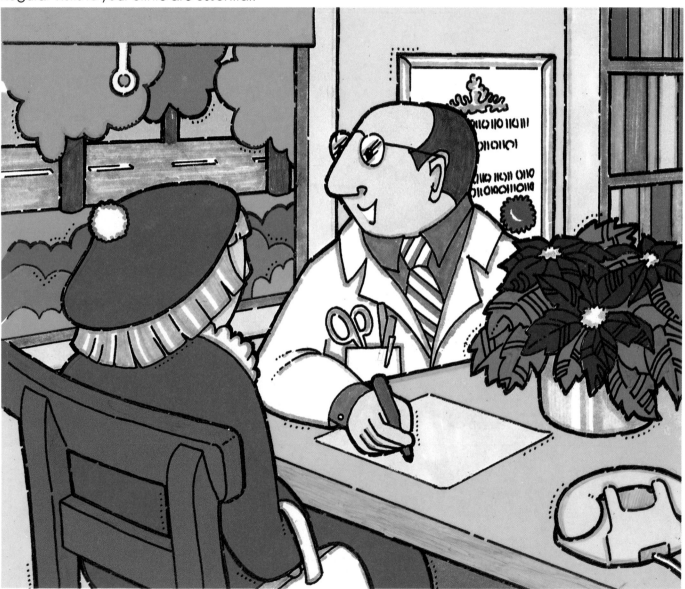

Summary

It must be stressed that the problems of long-term diabetes occur only in a minority of people with diabetes.

Remember:

- Good control of diabetes often prevents the development of these complications. Therefore, advice from regular clinic attendance is very important.
- Smoking accelerates arterial disease (affecting heart and feet), and may also have a bad effect on your eyes and kidneys.
- Obesity is often associated with arterial disease. Therefore, you should try to control your weight by an approved diet and exercise.

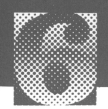

Diabetes and your daily life

Non-insulin dependent diabetes is, in the majority of cases, easily controlled by diet or tablets, and should therefore make very little difference to your daily life. Undoubtedly, the greatest change will be the need to modify and regulate your diet, but other day-to-day activities should be altered very little.

This chapter answers some of the most frequently asked questions about the influence of diabetes in your everyday activities, and discusses topics such as the financial implications of diabetes, and the additional steps you may need to take in order to remain fit and active.

Employment

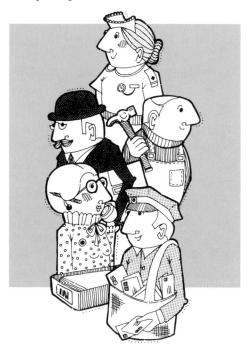

Diabetes and its influence on your work

For the vast majority of those with non-insulin dependent diabetes, their condition has no effect on their work. Consequently, your ability to function well should be as good as before you developed diabetes, perhaps even better. But there are certain careers in which having diabetes can prove a hindrance:

- If your work involves driving a Public Service Vehicle, and you have to take tablets for the treatment of your diabetes, then certain restrictions may be imposed (see 'Driving', page 77).
- Because of statutory regulations, you will not be allowed to fly aeroplanes.
- In some occupations, employers impose rather strict health regulations. For example, you cannot be accepted for entry into the Police Force, Armed Services or Fire Service, although if you are an established member you should be able to continue without difficulty.
- If you have a potentially highly dangerous job, e.g. deep-sea diving, steeple-jacking, or any job for which very high standards of fitness are required, you will probably have to change your occupation.

Diabetes and your employer

Unless you are employed in one of the occupations mentioned above, your employer need have no fears about your ability to continue employment or commence a new job. Unfortunately, some employers are not aware of the differences between insulin dependent diabetes and non-insulin dependent diabetes, and are therefore often reluctant to employ anybody with diabetes, in the mistaken belief that they might prove to be unreliable employees. Therefore, you should stress to your employer that with uncomplicated diabetes you are as capable of performing your job as a person without diabetes, and without risk to yourself or others. Shift work should pose no problems, and unlike those with insulin dependent diabetes, you do not require specific breaks for snacks or additional meals.

Occasionally, employers will not employ people with diabetes, because of their fear of future problems. In particular, they may be apprehensive that late complications may develop and render an employee incapable of full-time work.

Another frequently encountered problem, but one which usually can be overcome, is difficulty in negotiating superannuation arrangements, on account of the associated life insurance (see 'Life insurance', page 75).

If you experience difficulty in convincing your employer that you are fit to take up a new job, or to continue in your existing one, enlist the help of your GP, hospital doctor or the British Diabetic Association.

Only rarely should a person with diabetes need to be registered as disabled with the Disablement Resettlement Officer at the local Job Centre. However, should you develop serious complications, particularly loss of vision, you may find it helpful to register, and should not consider it a stigma to do so.

Financial implications of having diabetes

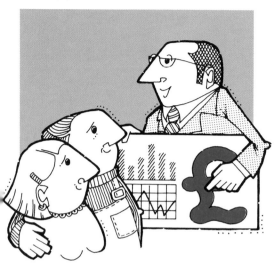

Insurance

Having diabetes should not give rise to any serious financial problems. All essential medical requirements are freely available on prescription under the National Health Service. Where you may experience increased expenditure, however, is in the field of life insurance. In all matters relating to insurance, it is essential to be completely frank with brokers or insurers, since concealment of any important medical facts may invalidate the insurance offered, with potentially serious financial and legal consequences.

Motor insurance

If you hold a motor insurance policy you must notify your insurance company or insurance broker that you have diabetes, as failure to do so may cause liability to be denied in the event of a claim. Most insurance companies will continue to offer cover to clients who develop diabetes, on receipt of a satisfactory medical certificate from their doctor. Attempts to impose an additional premium should be resisted.

New applicants for motor insurance may experience problems, but certain companies will quote normal rates, provided no accidents related to diabetes have occurred (there should be none in your case). If you encounter difficulties, details regarding brokers may be obtained from the British Diabetic Association.

Life insurance

Because of the possibility of long-term complications developing, it is normal for some loading to be placed on life and health insurance policies. If your diabetes is perfectly controlled and you have no complications, this loading should be small or non-existent but may be 5-10% on whole life policies. Loading for term assurance, e.g. mortgage protection or endowment policies, will be higher, but will normally be less than for those who are treated with insulin. If you experience any problems, you should seek help from the British Diabetic Association.

Sickness, accident and holiday insurance

It is <u>essential</u> that you declare your diabetes when taking out life or health insurance. Those with diabetes seeking personal sickness and accident insurance are likely to have to pay higher than normal premiums.

Those taking out insurance in connection with travel and holidays abroad must pay particular attention to the exclusion clauses which normally exclude all pre-existing illnesses. However, special cover for people with diabetes can usually be arranged, and the British Diabetic Association can give advice on this matter. Do not forget that failing to declare your diabetes when taking out travel insurance could nullify the policy.

Pensions/superannuation

Your pension rights should be unaffected by your diabetes. If you enter into a new scheme, it is essential that you declare your diabetes.

Other financial considerations

- Prescription charges in the UK are waived for all people with diabetes. A form (SP92) will be signed by your doctor, which will enable you to obtain an exemption certificate. This applies to all prescriptions, whether related to your diabetes or not.
- Your diet should not involve you in any additional expense. If, however, your expenditure has increased and this is creating difficulties, discussion with your local Social Security Office may enable you to obtain some help.
- Those who develop late complications, especially with their eyes, may be eligible for additional benefits.

Driving

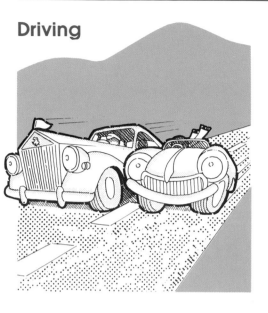

Points to remember

You must:
- Tell your insurance company that you have diabetes.
- Tell the licensing authorities (DVLC, Swansea SA99 1AT) that you have diabetes.

Applying for a driving licence

When you apply for a driving licence you have to answer one question of particular importance to you — Question 6(e) asks:

> "Have you now or have you ever had: epilepsy or sudden attacks of disabling giddiness or fainting or any mental illness or defect or any other disability which could affect your fitness as a driver either now or in the future?"

To this question you should answer 'Yes' whether you have diabetes treated with insulin, tablets, or diet alone. In the space provided for details, you should state that you have diabetes, adding that your diabetes is controlled by diet/tablets/insulin as appropriate. After you have completed and returned your application form, you may be sent a supplementary form, asking for further information, including the name and address of your doctor or hospital clinic, as well as your consent for the Driver and Vehicle Licensing Centre to approach your doctor for a detailed report on your diabetes. This complication of procedure does not mean that you will be refused a driving licence. The licence will normally be issued for three years and renewals will be made free of charge.

If your diabetes was diagnosed only recently and you already hold a 'life' licence, this will be revoked and replaced with a 'period' licence. Renewals can take several weeks, but should your licence pass its expiry date, you can continue to drive providing you have made application for a renewal.

Heavy Goods Vehicle (HGV) licences and Public Service Vehicle (PSV) licences are not prohibited to those with diabetes who do not take insulin, although some restrictions may be imposed on the Public Service Vehicle driver.

If you have non-insulin dependent diabetes controlled by diet alone, and have normal eyesight (with glasses if necessary), there are no special precautions which you need take. If however, you take tablets, you must ensure that you have your meals regularly, and should not drive if you are already late for a meal.

If you have any problems obtaining a driving licence, you should contact the British Diabetic Association.

Exercise and sport

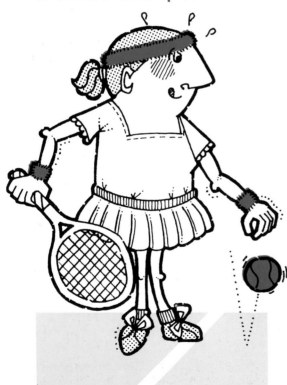

Exercise is an important aspect of the overall programme to control your diabetes. It not only lowers your blood sugar, but makes the action of insulin on your fat and muscle cells more efficient. Therefore, exercise is very beneficial, and there is no reason why you should not be able to continue heavy manual work or to enjoy any of the sports you played before your diabetes was diagnosed. There are leading tennis and badminton players, golfers, swimmers, cricketers, athletes and professional footballers who have diabetes.

Unlike a person with insulin dependent diabetes, there is no definite need for you to adjust your diet before strenuous exercise. If you are taking tablets, however, your blood sugar may fall lower than usual during exercise, but can be readily put right by an extra snack.

If you are a more sedentary type of person, not given to playing sport, you should, nonetheless, take routine, moderate exercise. Regular walking, for example, is better than short bursts of very strenuous exercise, and it can do much to preserve and even improve the circulation. A great deal of such mild exercise has to be taken to reduce weight, but it can make a contribution towards the general goal of weight control.

Fig. 6.1
Keeping fit is an essential aspect of maintaining good diabetic control.

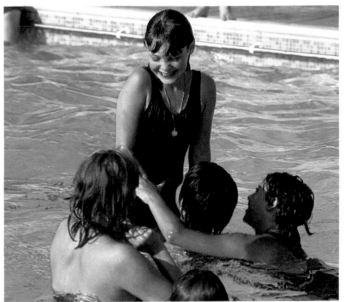

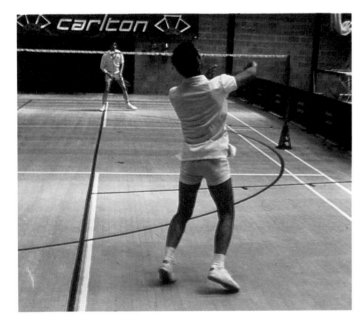

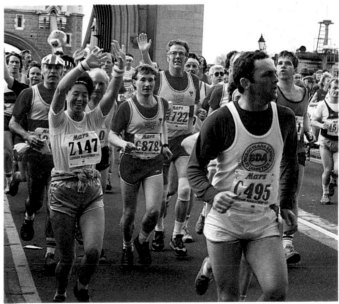

Retirement

All retired people have to adjust to the situation created by the cessation of the normal routine of going to work, and the fact that they are no longer associating with colleagues and work-mates. Loss of such contacts and interests may lead to bouts of depression, particularly in those who have never developed hobbies or interests outside their work. However, as long as you are otherwise fit, retirement should cause no greater problems for you than for anybody else.

If you are retired, it is essential that you should not allow your diabetes to stop you from developing new interests, or from making an active contribution to the community. For example, you could undertake voluntary work for the British Diabetic Association or other charitable organisations.

Do not forget to take advantage of the various Social Services available to you. Reduced fares on public transport and reduced entrance fees to certain places of entertainment, for example, could provide you with many opportunities not previously enjoyed.

Maintaining careful control of your diabetes, and taking whatever exercise is possible, are the best ways of ensuring that you remain healthy into old age.

Remember to ask your doctor or dietitian about adjustments to your diet if your activity increases or decreases.

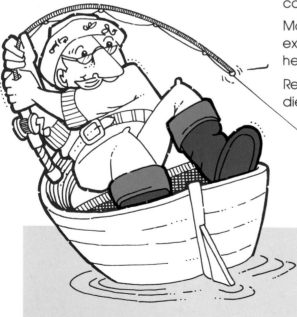
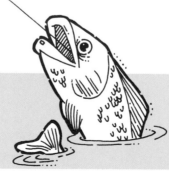

Fig. 6.2
Do not let your diabetes stop you
from enjoying a full and active
retirement.

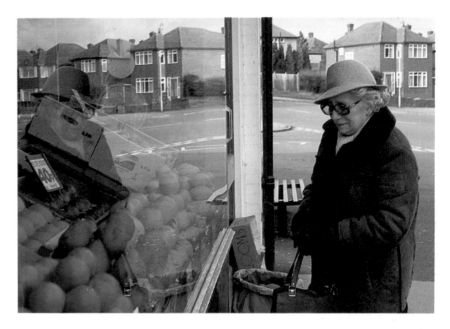

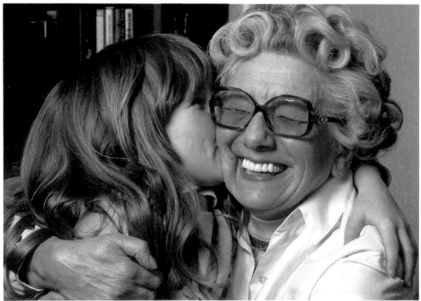

Travel and holidays

Your form of diabetes should not impose restrictions on travelling or holidays. It is wise, however, to take certain essential precautions, bearing in mind that even people without diabetes frequently suffer unforseen circumstances away from home.

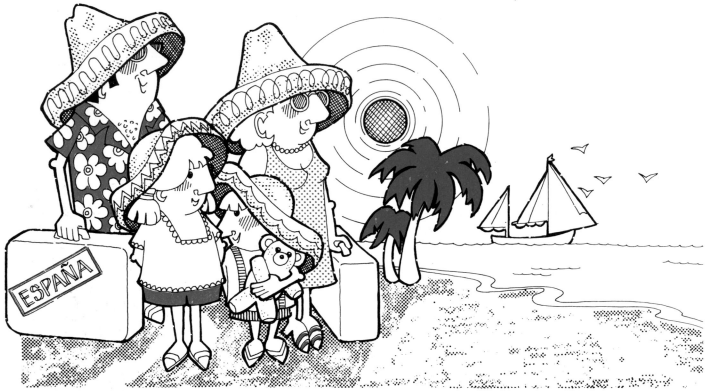

Illness

Mild gastroenteritis is an ailment commonly suffered while travelling abroad, and could cause your diabetes to go out of control temporarily (see 'Factors leading to loss of control', Chapter 4, page 61).

Whenever you feel unwell whilst travelling, test your urine. If the results show a high sugar reading, and you feel very dry and thirsty, consult a doctor. Most of the illnesses you are likely to experience while away from home will be mild and of short duration. Frequently, all you may notice are positive urine tests for a day or so, which then return to normal.

The most important points to remember when travelling at home or abroad are:

- Take your diabetes testing equipment with you.
- If on tablets, take more than you are likely to require. This is particularly important when travelling abroad, in case your return should be delayed.
- When travelling overseas, always take out health insurance.
- Always carry a card indicating that you have diabetes — this is essential if you take tablets.

Fig. 6.3
Always carry some form of identification.

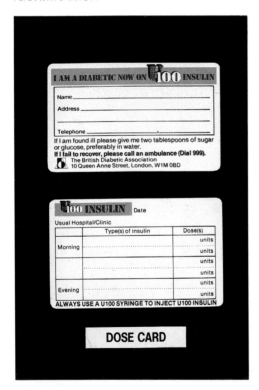

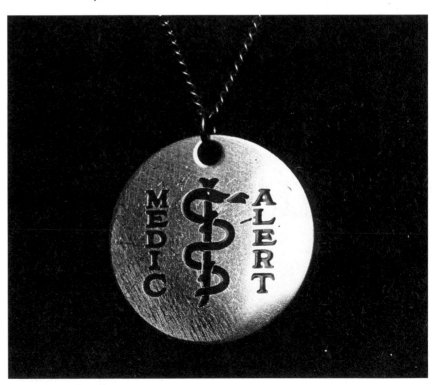

Foreign food

Eating different food, cooked in an unfamiliar way, may cause some problems, especially when eating out. Usually, though, you will find little difficulty in recognizing food similar to that of your normal diet.

An occasional deviation from your normal diet will do no real harm, and may merely cause an isolated positive urine test. If, however, you are overweight and have been on a diet, do not spoil all your prevous good work.

Air travel

You are not subject to any special restrictions, and you need take no special precautions.

Vaccination

Diabetes does not impose any restrictions on the vaccinations you may need if travelling abroad. However, immunization against certain illnesses may be followed by a day or so of feeling mildly unwell, together with a temporary rise in your blood sugar. This should cause you no concern.

Contraception, pregnancy, parenthood

Contraception

Because non-insulin dependent diabetes usually occurs in women who are middle-aged, contraception may not be a matter of concern. If, however, you are of appropriate age, then you should seek advice on contraception from your doctor or family planning clinic. Although the risk to a woman's health from the normal contraceptive pill is very slight, in your case your diabetes may increase this risk slightly. The contraceptive 'pill' may also lead to a rise in blood sugar, in which case some other form of contraception is advisable.

Fig. 6.4
Diabetes should not prevent you from getting married and having a family.

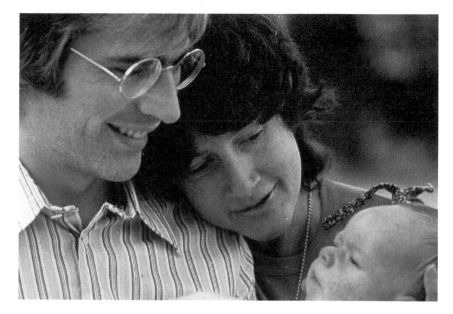

Pregnancy

If you are of child-bearing age and you intend having a child, you must take two important precautions:

1. You must ensure that your diabetes is well controlled when you are planning the pregnancy.

2. It is <u>absolutely essential</u> that once you know you are pregnant, you achieve perfect control and maintain it throughout pregnancy. The reason for this is that your growing baby, even though it will not have diabetes, will, nonetheless, be subject to your insulin and blood sugar levels.

Therefore, if you are planning a pregnancy, and certainly as soon as you become pregnant, you must report to your doctor and/or hospital clinic. Also, in order to make sure that your pregnancy continues without problems, you must regularly attend your diabetic clinic.

You may find that you require additional treatment during pregnancy, or even a period in hospital. Such special measures can usually be stopped, however, as soon as you have been delivered. With care by yourself and your doctor, a successful outcome is the rule rather than the exception.

Diabetes and heredity

The question asked by most parents is: "What are the chances of my child having diabetes?" There is no easy answer to this question, because the way in which diabetes is inherited is a complex process, which is not yet fully understood. In non-insulin dependent diabetes it does appear that inheritance plays a more significant role than in insulin dependent diabetes. But it must be stressed that it is most unlikely that any of your children will develop diabetes during childhood, as most inherited diabetes develops only later in life.

Many people who inherit the tendency to develop diabetes never actually do so. This is because other factors, including damage to the pancreas, emotional factors, obesity and, in some instances, even virus infections, are necessary for the development of diabetes.

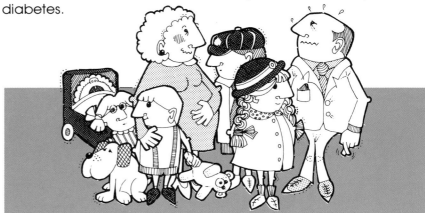

Diabetes and other illnesses

The effect of illness on diabetes

In the section on treatment (Chapter 4, page 61), it was indicated that under certain circumstances, such as illness or stress, your diabetes may go out of control temporarily. At such times, a few days loss of control is of no real significance, so long as you do not develop symptoms of thirst and dryness of the mouth, or pass large quantities of urine. If, however, these symptoms do occur, you must consult your doctor.

Diabetes and the treatment of other illnesses

Diabetes is no bar to the treatment — including operations — of any other disorder or illness.

Who is available to help?

With diet and tablets you should be able to control your diabetes. From time to time, however, you may develop problems about which you need specialized advice. On such occasions you may refer to a variety of individuals, including your doctor, nurses, dietitians, chiropodists, the Social Services and, of course, your local hospital clinic.

The British Diabetic Association

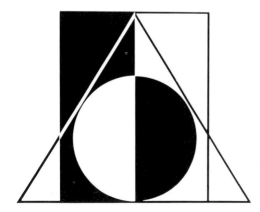

In spite of the help available to you from these specialist individuals and services, you may well have questions and problems relating to your day-to-day activities, such as careers, insurance, dietary problems etc. This is where the British Diabetic Association can be of great assistance. Through your local branch of the B.D.A. you will be able to meet others with diabetes. Such meetings can prove of immense value — particularly if your diabetes has only recently been diagnosed — in helping you to come to terms with the everyday problems of living with diabetes.

The British Diabetic Association is an independent registered charity. It was founded in 1934 to provide advice and help for those with diabetes, to overcome prejudice and ignorance about diabetes, and to raise money for research towards a cure.

The Association depends entirely on voluntary support — legacies, gifts and membership subscriptions. In 1939 there were 2,000 members; today there are over 100,000, but this represents little more than one tenth of the people with diabetes in the U.K.

Fig. 6.5
How the B.D.A. helps and supports those with diabetes.

Nation-wide organization
In the U.K., there are over 300 local branches, which hold regular meetings — all those with diabetes are welcome to attend.

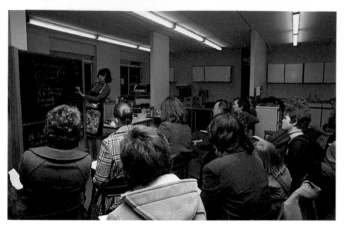

When you have problems
The B.D.A. will provide guidance and help on all problem affecting those with diabetes — but not individual treatment.

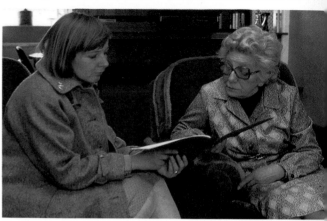

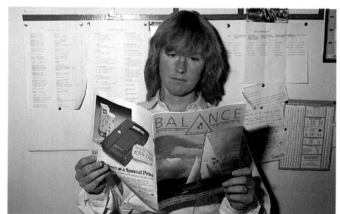

'Balance': a bi-monthly newspaper
Members receive 'Balance', the magazine of the B.D.A., free of charge, every two months. It reports progress in medical care and the latest news on legislation that affects those with diabetes. There is information on diets and recipes, articles on personalities and practical hints on day-to-day problems.

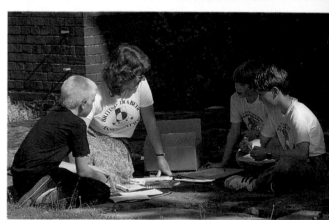

Holidays and advice for young people with diabetes
The Youth Department runs educational holidays for children with diabetes and adventure holidays for teenagers, both in the U.K. and abroad. This gives them the opportunity to learn to cope with their problems whilst taking part in normal activities without being the 'odd one out'. In addition, week-end teach ins, parents' meetings and International exchanges are a organised. Pen pals put in touch with each other. Advice is given on careers and other problems. Photo: Chris Schwarz

Liaison with Government Departments

The Association maintains close contact with Government Departments and other voluntary organizations, particularly where the elderly are concerned.

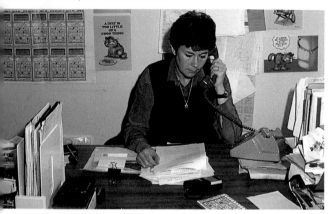

Holidays for adults with diabetes

Summer holidays are organized for adults with diabetes.

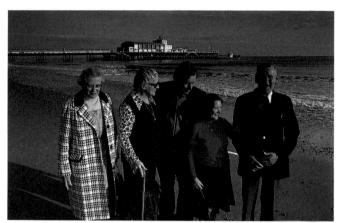

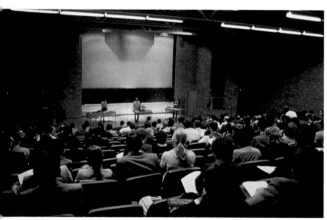

Conferences on diabetes

Through the B.D.A.'s Medical and Scientific, Educational and the Professional Services Sections, conferences are organized for all people concerned with diabetes, to ensure that they are kept abreast of advances in care and treatment. The B.D.A. is continually striving to make the life of people with diabetes easier and better in every way.

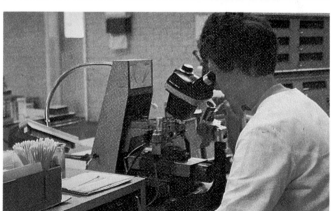

Research

One of the most important aspects of the B.D.A.'s work, certainly the most expensive, is research. The Association is the largest single contributor to diabetic research in the U.K., and currently supports some 65 research grants, totalling about £2m.

Some final comments on diabetes and your everyday life

- With relatively straightforward modifications to your daily life, effective control of your blood sugar level is possible.
- Adhere to your diet.
- If you have managed to lose weight, don't put it on again!
- If you need to take tablets, take them regularly.
- Take reasonable care of your general health, and your feet in particular.
- Attend your clinic for regular check-ups.

The late Dr R. D. Lawrence, physician and co-founder of the British Diabetic Association, wrote in his famous book 'The Diabetic Life':

> "There is no reason why a diabetic should not, if he can be taught to do so, lead a long and normal life. True, the diabetic life demands self-control from all its subjects, but it gives in return a full and active existence, with no real privations."

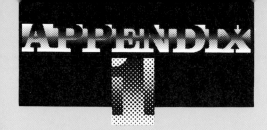

URINE TESTS

There are three reliable tests available in this country — Clinitest, Diastix and Diabur-Test 5000 (Fig. 4.3, page 60). Clinitest is slightly more sensitive and the colour change is easier to observe, but it does have the disadvantage that it requires the collection of a specimen of urine to put in a tube for testing. Diabur-Test 5000 and Diastix have the advantage that they are simpler to use, but if your sight is not perfect they may be less accurate.

There is a fourth test available, Clinistix, but this is not recommended, because it only tells you whether sugar is present or absent.

Urine tests provide a simple method of monitoring your blood sugar level, thereby helping you to maintain good control of your diabetes. When the blood sugar level rises beyond the renal threshold, sugar spills into the urine and will give rise to positive urine test results. Therefore, the aim of your treatment must be to make <u>all</u> your tests negative.

Clinitest

This test (Fig. 4.3a, page 60) requires the addition of urine to a tablet in a test tube and observing the colour change.

Equipment required

This includes:

- A test tube
- A dropper
- A container for urine
- Clinitest tablets.

Directions

1. Collect urine in a clean receptacle.

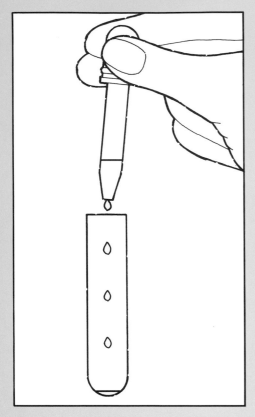

2. Draw urine into the dropper and place 5 drops into the test tube.

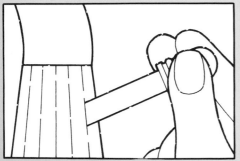

3. Rinse the dropper.

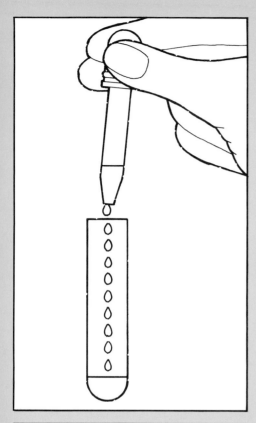

4. Draw water into the dropper and add 10 drops to the test tube.

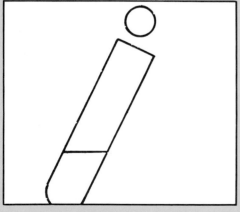

5. Drop one tablet into the test tube. Watch while the complete bubbling reaction takes place (see Interpretation of results, page 94). Do not shake the tube during the reaction, nor for 15 seconds after the bubbling has stopped.

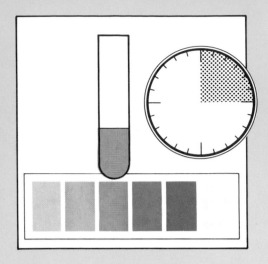

6. After the 15 seconds waiting period, shake the test tube gently and compare the colour of the liquid with the colour chart provided and note down the per cent result.

Note: For accurate results, always use special Clinitest droppers and test tubes, which can be obtained from your pharmacy.

Interpretation of the results

NEGATIVE — no sugar (glucose)

The liquid will be blue at the end of the waiting period of 15 seconds. The whitish sediment that may form has no bearing on the test and should be ignored.

POSITIVE — sugar present

The more sugar in the urine, the greater the colour change and the more rapidly it occurs. The amount of sugar is determined by comparing the colour of the solution in the test tube with the colour chart, at the end of the 15 second waiting period. Colour changes developing after the 15 second waiting period should be disregarded.

IMPORTANT

It is essential that you carefully observe the solution in the test tube while the bubbling reaction takes place and during the 15 second waiting period, in order to detect the rapid 'pass-through' colour changes. If the colours rapidly pass through green, tan and orange to a dark greenish-brown, you should record the result as over 2% sugar, without comparing the final colour development with the colour chart.

The colour chart and the above instructions must be used with Clinitest Reagent Tablets only.

Care and handling of Clinitest Reagent Tablets

- Keep tablets away from direct heat and sunlight (but not in a refrigerator).

- Replace bottle cap <u>immediately</u> after removing the tablet and before starting the test, since the tablets absorb moisture and spoil (turning dark blue) if the bottle is not kept tightly closed.

- Handle tablets cautiously; they contain caustic soda.

Diastix

Diastix (Fig. 4.3b page 60) involves placing a strip of special paper in the stream of urine and then observing the colour change.

Equipment required

This test requires Diastix strips only.

Directions

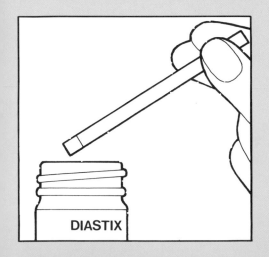

1. Remove test strip from the bottle and replace the cap promptly and tightly.

    It is important that you:
    - <u>Do not touch</u> the test area of the strip.
    - Use <u>only</u> the reagent strips with the <u>pale blue test areas</u> (similar in colour to the 'negative' colour block of the colour chart on the bottle label).
    - Do not remove the small packet of moisture – absorbing crystals from the bottle.

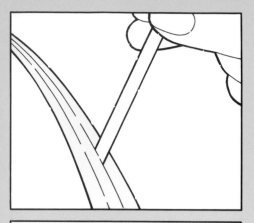

2. Dip the reagent strip into the stream of urine for 2 seconds and remove.

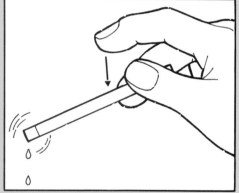

3. Tap the edge of the strip to remove excess urine.

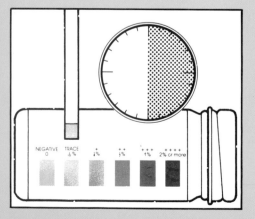

4. Wait 30 seconds and then immediately compare the colour of the test area against the Diastix colour chart, which ranges from 0% (blue) to 2% or more (brown). Record the result.

Note If you are using Keto-Diastix ignore the strips with the buff coloured test area, which are used for the measurement of ketones.

Diabur-Test 5000

The procedure with Diabur-Test 5000 (Fig. 43c, page 60) is similar to that for Diastix.

Equipment required

Diabur-Test 5000 test strips.

Directions

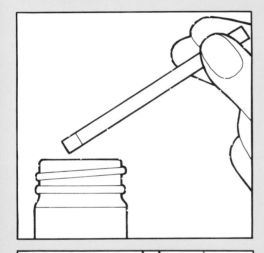

1. Remove a strip from the container.

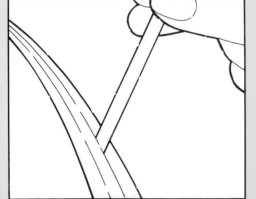

2. Briefly dip the strip into the stream of urine or specimen.

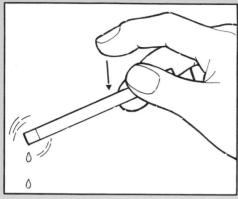

3. Shake off the excess urine.

4. Wait 2 minutes.

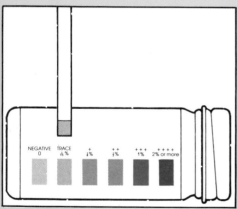

5. Compare the colour of the test area with the Diabur colour scale and record the result.

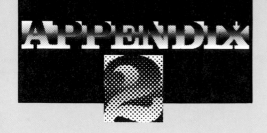

FOOD VALUES FOR THOSE WITH DIABETES

The first column in the following tables, with the exception of Tables II and VII, lists foods that provide 10 grams of carbohydrate when eaten in the amount stated. The amount is described in either of two ways:

1. A weight measured in grams (g)
2. A spoon measure.

If using the spoon measures, use standard kitchen measuring spoons, as used in compiling this list. The tablespoon (tbsp) measurement is based on a 15ml spoon, the teaspoon (tsp) on a 5ml spoon (all are level spoonsful).

Each item of food, if eaten in the amount stated (either the gram weight or spoon measure), will provide 10 grams of carbohydrate, i.e. 1 'exchange', 1 'portion' or 1 'line'.

For the overweight, the energy (calorie) intake is most important, and therefore the calorie content of each serving of food is given in the third column.

It is generally recommended that at least half of your carbohydrate allowance should come from the foods listed in the tables for starch (Table I) and vegetables (TABLES V and X). Also, the foods marked with an asterisk are all good (*) or very good (* *) sources of fibre, and it is recommended that you include as many of these as possible in your diet each day.

WEIGHTS AND MEASURES

Most diet scales are marked in metric weights, i.e. grams, and we recommend that you use this scale if weighing. If you only have scales marked in imperial weights, i.e. pounds and ounces, the following conversion charts may be useful:

Grams (g)		Approx. ounces
25	=	1
50	=	2
75	=	3
100	=	4
150	=	5
175	=	6
200	=	7

Millilitres (ml)		Approx. pints
75	=	$\frac{1}{8}$
150	=	¼
275	=	½
425	=	¾
550	=	1

TABLE I	Starchy foods
TABLE II	Bread
TABLE III	Breakfast cereals
TABLE IV	Biscuits, crackers, crispbreads
TABLE V	Vegetables
TABLE VI	Fruits
TABLE VII	Vegetables and some fruits
TABLE VIII	Fruit juices
TABLE IX	Processed foods
TABLE X	Milk and milk products
TABLE XI	Low-carbohydrate, high-calorie foods
TABLE XII	Alcoholic drinks

TABLE I

STARCHY FOODS	Approximate measure	Approximate weight of food (g) containing 10g carbohydrate	Calorie content
Arrowroot/custard powder/cornflour	1 tbsp	10	35
Barley, raw	1 tbsp	10	40
Flour, plain, white	1½ tbsp	10	40
Flour, self-raising, white	1½ tbsp	10	45
* Flour, wholemeal, wholewheat	2 tbsp	15	50
**Oats, uncooked	3 tbsp	15	60
Spaghetti, white, uncooked	6 long (19") strands	10	45
**Spaghetti, wholewheat, uncooked	20 short (10") strands	15	50
* Spaghetti/macaroni, cooked	2 tbsp	10	45
Rice, white, uncooked	1 tbsp	10	45
**Rice, brown, uncooked	1 tbsp	10	40
Sago/tapioca/semolina, uncooked	2 tsp	10	35
* Soya flour, full fat	14 tbsp	75	300
* Soya flour, low fat	9 tbsp	50	125
* Soya granules, dry	13 tbsp	75	200

* Good fibre content
** Very good fibre content

TABLE II

BREAD	Size of loaf	Type of bread	Approximate weight of carbohydrate (g)	Calorie content
1 thin slice	small	wholemeal*	10	50
1 thin slice	small	white	10	50
1 thin slice	large	wholemeal*	13	69
1 thin slice	large	white	15	75
1 thick slice	large	wholemeal*	20	100
1 thick slice	large	white	26	125
1 roll		wholemeal*	13	69
1 roll		white	15	75

*Good fibre content

TABLE III

BREAKFAST CEREALS	Approximate measure	Approximate weight of food (g) containing 10g carbohydrate	Calorie content
**Allbran	5 tbsp	20	50
**Bran Buds	4 tbsp	20	50
Cornflakes	5 tbsp	10	40
**Muesli (unsweetened)	2 tbsp	15	50
**Muesli (sweetened)	2 tbsp	15	55
**Puffed Wheat	15 tbsp	15	50
Rice Krispies	6 tbsp	10	40
**Shredded Wheat	2/3 of one		80
Special K	8 tbsp	15	50
**Spoonsize Cubs	12-14		45
**Weetabix	1		60
**Weetaflakes	4 tbsp	15	50

**Very good fibre content

Values for all individual breakfast cereals are given in 'Countdown'.

TABLE IV

BISCUITS, CRACKERS, CRISPBREADS	Approximate measure	Approximate weight of food (g) containing 10g carbohydrate	Calorie content
Biscuits, plain	2	15	60
**Biscuits, digestive or wholemeal	1	15	70
Biscuits, cream or chocolate	1	10	60
Crackers, plain	2	15	70
Crispbread	2	15	50

**Good fibre content

Values for individual biscuits are given in 'Countdown'.

TABLE V

VEGETABLES+	Approximate measure	Approximate weight of food (g) containing 10g carbohydrate	Calorie content
**Beans, baked	4 tbsp	75	55
**Beans, broad, boiled	10 tbsp	150	75
**Beans, dried, all types, raw	2 tbsp	20	55
*Beetroot, cooked, whole	2 small	100	45
*Lentils, dry, raw	2 tbsp	20	60
*Onions, raw	1 large	200	45
*Parsnips, raw	1 small	90	45
*Peas, marrow fat or processed	7 tbsp	75	60
*Peas, dried, all types, raw	2 tbsp	20	60
*Plantain, green, raw, peeled	small slice	35	40
*Potatoes, raw	1 small egg-sized	50	45
*Potatoes, boiled	1 small egg-sized	50	40
*Potatoes, chips (weighed when cooked)	4-5 chips	25	65
**Potatoes, jacket (weighed with skin)	1 small-sized	50	45
*Potatoes, mashed	1 small scoop	50	80
*Potatoes, roast	½ medium-sized	40	65
*Sweetcorn, canned or frozen	5 tbsp	60	45
**Sweetcorn, on the cob	½ medium cob	75	60
*Sweet potato, raw, peeled	1 small slice	50	45

* Good fibre content
** Very good fibre content
+ Vegetables which can be eaten freely are listed in TABLE X

TABLE VI

FRUITS+	Approximate measure	Approximate weight of food (g) containing 10g carbohydrate	Calorie content
*Apples, eating, whole	1 medium	110	50
*Apples, cooking, whole	1 medium	125	55
*Apples, stewed without sugar	6 tbsp	125	40
*Apricots, fresh, whole	3 medium	160	40
*Apricots, dried, raw	4 small	25	45
*Bananas, whole	5½" in length	90	40
*Bananas, peeled	3½" in length	50	40
*Bilberries, raw	5 tbsp	75	40
*Blackberries, raw	10 tbsp	150	45
*Blackcurrants, raw	10 tbsp	150	45
*Cherries, fresh, whole	12 tbsp	100	40
*Currants, dried	2 tbsp	15	35
*Damsons, raw, whole	7	120	40
*Dates, fresh, whole	3 medium	50	40
*Dates, dried, without stones	3 small	15	40
*Figs, fresh, whole	1	100	40
*Figs, dried	1	20	45
*Grapes, whole	10 large	75	40
*Grapefruit, whole	1 very large	400	45
*Greengages, fresh, whole	5	90	40
*Guavas, fresh, peeled	1	70	45
*Mango, fresh, whole	⅓ of a large one	100	40

FRUITS+	Approximate measure	Approximate weight of food (g) containing 10g carbohydrate	Calorie content
Melon, all types, weighed with skin	large slice	300	40
*Nectarine, fresh, whole	1	90	40
*Orange, fresh, whole	1 large	150	40
*Pawpaw, fresh, whole	$\frac{1}{6}$ of a large one	80	50
*Peach, fresh, whole	1 large	125	40
*Pears, fresh, whole	1 large	130	40
*Pineapple, fresh, no skin or core	1 thick slice	90	40
*Plums, cooking, fresh, whole	4 medium	180	40
*Plums, dessert, fresh, whole	2 large	110	40
*Pomegranate, fresh, whole	1 small	110	40
*Prunes, dried, without stones	2 large	25	40
*Raisins, dried	2 tbsp	15	35
*Raspberries, fresh	12 tbsp	175	45
*Strawberries, fresh	15 medium	160	40
*Sultanas, dried	2 tbsp	15	40
*Tangerines, fresh, whole	2 large	175	40

* Good fibre content

+ A few fruits contain very little natural sugar and can be taken in generous helpings without counting calories, e.g. cranberries, gooseberries, lemons, loganberries and rhubarb — all other fruits should be counted into your diet.

TABLE VII

VEGETABLES AND SOME FRUITS

The following foods contain no more than 5g of carbohydrate and 20—25 calories in a normal (approximately 100g/ 4oz) serving:

VEGETABLES

*Artichokes, cooked	*Lettuce
*Asparagus, cooked	*Marrow, cooked
*Aubergine, cooked	*Mushrooms, raw
*Beans, fresh runner	Mustard and cress
*Beansprouts, raw	Okra, raw
*Broccoli	*Onions, boiled
**Brussels sprouts	Peppers
**Cabbage, raw	*Pumpkin
**Carrots, cooked	Radishes
*Cauliflower, cooked	Spinach, boiled
**Celery, raw or cooked	*Swede, boiled
*Courgettes	*Tomatoes, raw and canned
*Cucumber	*Turnip
**Leeks, cooked	Watercress

REMEMBER: White sauces count!

FRUITS

Cranberries	Loganberries	Melon
*Currants, red and black	Grapefruit (½)	*Raspberries
Gooseberries	Lemons	Rhubarb

*Good fibre content
**Very good fibre content

TABLE VIII

FRUIT JUICES+	Approximate measure	Approximate weight of food (g) containing 10g carbohydrate	Calorie content
Apple juice, unsweetened	6 tbsp	85	40
Blackcurrant, unsweetened	7 tbsp	100	40
Grapefruit, unsweetened	8 tbsp	125	45
Orange, unsweetened	7 tbsp	100	40
Pineapple, unsweetened	6 tbsp	85	40
Tomato, unsweetened	1 large glass	275	50

+The carbohydrate value will vary slightly according to the time of year.

TABLE IX

PROCESSED FOODS+	Approximate measure	Approximate weight of food (g) containing 10g carbohydrate	Calorie content
FOODS			
Beefburgers, frozen	3 small	—	450
Canned soup	½ medium tin (thick)	—	170
Fish fingers	2	—	110
Complan	3 tbsp	—	
Ice-cream	1 scoop	—	90
Sausages	2 thick	110	400
Scotch egg	½	—	180
DRINKS			
Beer, draught	½ pint		100
Lager, draught	¾ pint		135
Cider, dry	¾ pint		120
Cider, sweet	½ pint		95
Cider, vintage	¼ pint		75

+ This table lists a few typical foods and drinks which provide approximately 10g of carbohydrate. As there are considerable variations between the products marketed by different manufacturers, it is recommended that if your family uses processed foods regularly, you should refer to the comprehensive lists of manufactured foods and alcoholic drinks provided in 'Countdown'.

TABLE X

MILK AND MILK PRODUCTS	Approximate measure	Approximate weight of food (g) containing 10g carbohydrate	Calorie content
Milk, fresh	1 cup	200	130
Milk, fresh, semi-skimmed	1 cup	200	95
Milk, fresh, skimmed	1 cup	200	70
Milk, dried, whole	8 tsps	25	125
Milk, dried, skimmed	10 tsps	20	70
Milk, evaporated	6 tblsp	90	145
Yoghurt, plain, low fat	1 small carton	150	80

TABLE XI

LOW-CARBOHYDRATE, HIGH-CALORIE FOODS +	Approximate measure	Approximate weight of food (g)	Calorie content
DAIRY PRODUCTS			
Butter/margarine	5 tsp	25	185
Low fat spreads	5 tsp	25	95
Egg — medium uncooked	1	55	80
Cream, single	Small pot	150	320
Cream, double	Small pot	150	670
Cream, whipped	Small pot	150	500
Cheese, Cheddar	Small matchbox size	25	100
Cheese, cottage	5 tbsp	100	110
Cheese, cream	1 heaped tbsp	25	110
Cheese, Edam	Small matchbox size	25	75
Cheese, Parmesan	3 tbsp	25	100
Cheese, Quark	Small pot	100	90
Cheese, Stilton	Small matchbox size	25	115
Cheese spread	3 tbsp	50	140
MEAT			
Bacon, lean, grilled	1 rasher	25	75
Bacon, lean, fried	1 rasher	25	80
Bacon, streaky, grilled	1 rasher	25	105
Bacon, streaky, fried	1 rasher	25	125
Meat, lean, raw	1 av. helping	100	125
Meat, lean, cooked	1 av. helping	100	160
Meat, fatty, raw	1 av. helping	100	410
Poultry, white meat, cooked	1 av. helping	100	140
Poultry, dark meat, cooked	1 av. helping	100	155
Lamb, cutlet, grilled	1 medium	100	250
Pork chop, grilled	1 medium	150	390
Corned beef	2 slices	50	110

LOW-CARBOHYDRATE, HIGH-CALORIE FOODS	Approximate measure	Approximate weight of food (g)	Calorie content
FISH			
Fish fillets, white, raw	1 av. helping	100	80
Fish fillets, oily, raw	1 av. helping	100	230
Shellfish, shelled	1 av. helping	100	80-100
NUTS			
Almonds, shelled	4 tbsp	50	280
Brazil, shelled	14 medium	50	310
Hazelnuts, shelled	6 tbsp	50	190
Coconut, dried	5 tbsp	25	150
Peanuts, roast	1 small packet	25	145
Walnuts	16 halves	50	130
MISCELLANEOUS			
Oil, vegetable	1 tbsp	15	135
Suet, shredded	6 tbsp	50	420

+NOTE: Because the foods and drinks listed in TABLE XI contain a high calorie content, particular care is required if you are overweight.

TABLE XII

The carbohydrate and/or calorie content of a range of alcoholic drinks is listed below. If you are on insulin or large doses of oral hypoglycaemic agents you are reminded **NOT** to exchange alcohol for 'food exchanges' (portions). Providing you do not exceed recommended amount of 3 drinks a day (see page 54) the carbohydrate contribution can be ignored. We do not advise you to drink beers or lager/ciders that exceed an alcohol content of 5%.

Alcoholic drinks		Approximate measure	Carbohydrate (g)	Calorie content
Beer		per ½ pint	10	100/130
Cider, dry		per ½ pint	5	100
sweet		per ½ pint	10	100/120
Lager		per ½ pint	7-10	85/110
Vermouth, dry		1 pub measure (⅓ gill)	1-5	50/60
sweet		1 pub measure (⅓ gill)	5-10	70/80
Sherry, dry		1 pub measure (⅓ gill)	1-2	50/60
sweet		1 pub measure (⅓ gill)	5-10	70/90
Sparkling wine/Champagne	dry	4 fl oz/113ml glass	1-2	80/90
	sweet	4 fl oz/113ml glass	5-10	90/100
Wine (red/white)	dry	4 fl oz/113ml glass	1-2	70/80
	sweet	4 fl oz/113ml glass	5-10	80/100
Spirits, i.e. whisky, gin, rum, vodka, brandy, advocaat		1 pub measure ($\frac{1}{6}$ gill)	neg	50/70
Liqueurs		1 pub measure ($\frac{1}{6}$ gill)	5-10	80/100

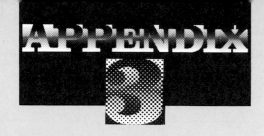

B.D.A. PUBLICATIONS

Children's books

I HAVE DIABETES

A booklet in the popular Althea series for children and parents which explains diabetes as a story.
Colour illustrations

Diet and recipe books

BETTER COOKERY FOR DIABETICS

by BDA dietitian, Jill Metcalfe. Over 130 delicious and healthy recipes with practical hints for following the low fat, high fibre diet recommended for diabetics. Spiral bound, 16 pages of colour illustrations.

COOKING THE NEW DIABETIC WAY — THE HIGH FIBRE, CALORIE-CONSCIOUS COOKBOOK

compiled by BDA dietitian Jill Metcalfe. Over 260 low fat, reduced calories, high fibre recipes. A useful book for diabetics who need to lose weight. Recipes feature servings for two and four. Eight pages of colour illustrations.

VEGETARIAN ON A DIET

the high fibre, low sugar, low fat, wholefood vegetarian cook book by Margaret Cousins and Jill Metcalfe. An introduction to the benefits of the vegetarian way of eating with specific advice for the diabetic and weight watcher. Featuring a wide range of exciting but practical recipes with an extensive wholefood food values list. All recipes have complete carbohydrate and calorie counts.

COUNTDOWN

A guide to the carbohydrate and calorie content of manufactured foods and drinks.
Designed to help you choose your food wisely.

SIMPLE DIABETIC COOKERY

A booklet of 50 one and two serving high fibre recipes.

SIMPLE HOME BAKING

A booklet of 50 high fibre, reduced fat home baking recipes including cakes, biscuits and breads. The recipes range from basic bread to celebration cakes and all are carbohydrate and calorie calculated.

Educational books

DIABETES EXPLAINED

by Dr Arnold Bloom (4th edition). Provides a clear explanation of diabetes and its successful management. Hard cover.

LIFE WITH DIABETES

by Dr Arnold Bloom. Illustrated booklet which takes a practical look at diabetes.

GLOSSARY

Acidosis
A build-up of acids, usually ketones, in the blood.

Acetone
Is a sweet smelling ketone that may be smelt on the breath of people with ketones in the blood.

Adrenalin
Is the hormone released from the central portion of the adrenal glands in response to a stress or emergency, e.g. an illness, a hypoglycaemic reaction, a fright.

Albumen
A blood protein, which may appear in the urine when the kidneys are damaged.

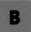

Beta cells
The cells of the islets of Langerhans in the pancreas that produce insulin.

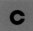

Calorie
A standard measurement of heat or energy used to assess the energy value of food. It is being replaced by the kilojoule.
1 calorie = 4.2 kilojoules.

Carbohydrate (CHO)
A class of foodstuff that is an important source of energy to the body. It is mainly represented by sugars and starches.

Cataract
An opacity in the lens of the eye that may be caused by long-standing diabetes.

Coma
A state of unconsciousness. In diabetes this can result from severe hypoglycaemia or severe keto-acidosis.

Cortisol

A hormone released from the outer portion of the adrenal glands during stress, shock, infection, etc.

Dehydration

Refers to being depleted of water. It occurs when the blood sugar is high for long periods, as in keto-acidosis.

Dextrose

Simply sugar (see glucose).

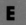

Electrolytes

A term applied to the important salts of the body, such as sodium, potassium, chlorides and bicarbonate.

Enuresis

Involuntary passage of urine, bedwetting.

Exchange diet

One in which a fixed number of servings of carbohydrate, fat, protein and milk foods is prescribed so as to control total energy intake as well as the quantities of all major foodstuffs.

Fat atrophy

Disappearance of fat from under the skin, at the site of insulin injection. More common with less refined insulins.

Fat hypertrophy

Swelling of the fat where insulin is being injected.

Fatty acids

These are the main components of body fat in which they are combined with glycerol (glycerine).

Fructose

A sugar occurring in fruit, a simple carbohydrate.

Gangrene

Death of tissue due to poor blood supply.

Glucose

Simple sugar.

Glucagon

A hormone produced by cells of the islets of Langerhans in the pancreas. It tends to raise the blood sugar level.

Gluconeogenesis

The making of glucose by the liver, especially from protein breakdown products.

Glycogen

Is made by the body from glucose and is the main complex CHO in animals. It is stored in the liver and muscles.

Glycogenolysis

The process of releasing glucose from glycogen stored in the liver.

Glycosuria

The presence of sugar in the urine.

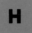

Haemoglobin A, (glycosylated haemoglobin)

A test used to assess long-term diabetic control.

Hormone

The name given to a chemical substance released by an organ into the bloodstream. Hormones are responsible for controlling such functions as metabolism, growth, sex development, blood sugar levels, etc.

Hyperglycaemia

A high blood sugar.

Hypoglycaemia or 'hypo'

A low blood sugar (less than 3 mmol/l).

Insulin

A hormone produced by the beta cells in the islets of Langerhans in the pancreas. It enables glucose in the blood to get into the cells and be used for energy or to be stored.

Insulin reaction

Another term for hypoglycaemic reaction.

Intestine

The gut or bowel between the stomach and the anus.

Intravenous glucose

This is glucose that is injected directly into a vein.

Intravenous infusion

Liquid, such as water containing salt and glucose, being slowly injected, usually out of a bottle and over a long period of time, directly into the bloodstream via a vein.

Keto-acidosis or ketosis

A state of overproduction of ketones in the body which causes a build-up of acids in the blood.

Ketones

When fats are broken down in the body, ketones are produced. If a lot of fat is broken down, as in poorly controlled diabetes, the ketones accumulate in the blood, pass into the urine and can be smelt on the breath.

Ketonuria

The presence of ketones in the urine.

L

Lactose
The sugar found in milk.

Lipolysis
Breakdown of fat caused by starvation or lack of insulin.

M

Metabolism
The system of chemical control in the body.

Ml
Millilitre, a measure of volume.

mmol/l
Millimole per litre, a measure of the concentration of a substance.

N

Neuropathy
A disorder of the nerves, where the signals in them are not properly conducted. It is sometimes seen in those with diabetes.

O

Ophthalmologist
An eye specialist.

P

Pancreas
A long organ lying across the back of the abdomen. Part of it secretes digestive juices into the intestine, but its islets of Langerhans, pinpoint sized collections of cells scattered throughout it like currants in a cake, secrete insulin and glucagon.

Polydipsia
Excessive thirst.

Polyuria
The passing of large quantities of urine, and in diabetes caused

when there is overflow into the urine of excess glucose from the bloodstream.

Portion

One portion equals 10 grams of carbohydrate in this book.

Portion diet

One in which only the carbohydrate-containing foods are carefully prescribed in quantity in terms of 'portions'.

Post-prandial

After the meal.

Protein

A major food component important in body building, but may provide energy.

Reaction

See hypoglycaemia

Renal threshold

The level of sugar in the blood above which it spills over into the urine.

Retina

The light-receptive layer at the back of the eye. It is an extension of the optic nerve in the eye.

Retinopathy

Damage to the retina. May be caused by long-standing diabetes.

Sorbitol

A sweetening agent which when absorbed is converted in the liver to fructose.

Sucrose

Cane sugar.

Thrush

A fungal infection of nails, skin, mouth or vagina.

Triglyceride

A combination of fats used to carry or store fats in the body.

Unit

Refers to a quantity chosen as a standard basic measurement of insulin.

Vitamins

Compounds found in small quantities in natural foods. They are required for normal growth and maintenance of life, although they do not themselves provide energy or substance.

INDEX

P

Pancreas, 14
Pancreatic disease causing diabetes, 7
Pasta, 42
Pensions, 76
Pill, The, see Contraceptive pill
Portions see Exchanges
Potatoes, 29
Pregnancy, 85-86
Prescription charges, 76
Processed foods, 110
Protein
    foods containing, 24, 31, 46
    metabolism, 13

R

Rations see Exchanges
Renal threshold of blood sugar, 17, 91
Research into diabetes, 89
Retinal damage, 67
Retirement, 80-81
Rice, wholegrain, 42

S

Seasonings, 47
Shoes, 65-66
Sickness insurance, 76
    see also Illness
Snacks, 34
Social life, 78-84
    eating out, 34, 51-52
    retirement, 80-81
Social Security help, 76
Sports see Exercise
Starchy foods, 101
Stress causing loss of control, 62

Sugar
    blood see Blood sugar
    conversion to energy, 4, 12
    intake control, 22
    in urine see Glycosuria
        testing for see urine tests
    metabolism, 12
    substitutes, 34, 47, 49
Sulphonylurea, 54, 55
Superannuation, 76
Sweeteners, 34, 47, 49
Symptoms
    diabetes, 9
    hyperglycaemia, 17-19

T

Tablets, 22
    lack of response to, 62
    side effects, 56-57
    treatment queries, 55-56
    when to use, 54
    which to use, 54
Thirst, 18, 62
Thrush, 18
Tiredness, 18
Toenail cutting, 65
Travel, 82-84
Travel insurance, 76
Treatment of diabetes, 21-56
    effectiveness of, 57-62

U

Urine
    excess passing of, 17
    sugar in, 17-18